New Frontiers in Hip Arthroscopy

Editors

MARIO HEVESI
SHANE J. NHO

CLINICS IN SPORTS MEDICINE

www.sportsmed.theclinics.com

Consulting Editor
F. WINSTON GWATHMEY

October 2026 • Volume 45 • Number 4

ELSEVIER

1818 Market Street • Suite 3323 • Philadelphia, Pennsylvania, 19103-2899

http://www.theclinics.com

CLINICS IN SPORTS MEDICINE Volume 45, Number 4
October 2026 ISSN 0278-5919, ISBN-13: 978-0-443-41586-9

Editor: Megan Ashdown
Developmental Editor: Malvika Shah

Publishing Office: *Clinics in Sports Medicine* (ISSN 0278-5919) is published quarterly by Elsevier Inc., 1818 Market Street, Philadelphia, PA 19103, United States. Periodicals postage paid at New York, NY and additional mailing offices. USA POSTMASTER: Send address changes to *Clinics in Sports Medicine*, Elsevier Customer Service Department, 3251 Riverport Lane, Maryland Heights, MO 63043, USA. Months of issue are January, April, July, and October. Subscription prices are $399.00 per year (US individuals), $100.00 per year (US students), $443.00 per year (Canadian individuals), $100.00 (Canadian students), $519.00 per year (foreign individuals), and $235.00 per year (foreign students). For institutional access pricing please contact Customer Service via the contact information below. Foreign air speed delivery is included in all *Clinics* subscription prices. All prices are subject to change without notice. Orders, claims, and journal inquiries: Please visit our Support Hub page https://service.elsevier.com for assistance.

Reprints. For copies of 100 or more of articles in this publication, please contact the Commercial Reprints Department, Elsevier Inc., 360 Park Avenue South, New York, NY 10010-1710. Tel.: 212-633-3874; Fax: 212-633-3820; E-mail: reprints@elsevier.com.

Clinics in Sports Medicine is covered in *MEDLINE/PubMed (Index Medicus) Current Contents/Clinical Medicine, Excerpta Medica,* and *ISI/Biomed.*

Contributors

CONSULTING EDITOR

F. WINSTON GWATHMEY, MD
Associate Professor of Orthopaedic Surgery, University of Virginia Health System, Charlottesville, Virginia, USA; Vice Chair for Orthopaedic Education and Residency Program Director, Team Physician, UVA and JMU Athletics, Charlottesville, Virginia, USA

EDITORS

MARIO HEVESI, MD, PhD
Associate Professor of Orthopedic Surgery, Department of Orthopedic Surgery and Sports Medicine, Mayo Clinic, Rochester, Minnesota, USA

SHANE J. NHO, MD, MS
Professor, Department of Orthopedic Surgery, Surgeon, Section of Young Adult Hip Surgery, Division of Sports Medicine, Midwest Orthopaedics at Rush, Rush University Medical Center, Chicago, Illinois, USA

AUTHORS

ZACHARY S. AMAN, MD
Resident, Department of Orthopedic Surgery, Duke University Medical Center, Durham, North Carolina, USA

NEEL BADHE, BA
Student, School of Clinical Medicine, University of Cambridge, Cambridge, United Kingdom

KRISTEN I. BARTON, MD, PhD, FRCSC
Fellow, Section of Young Adult Hip Surgery, Division of Sports Medicine, Department of Orthopedic Surgery, Rush University Medical Center, Chicago, Illinois, USA

ALEXANDRIA CHRUMKA, MD
Fellow Physician, Department of Orthopedic Surgery, University of Wisconsin-Madison, Madison, Wisconsin, USA

EMMETT J. CLEARY, MD
Resident Physician, Department of Orthopedic Surgery, Mayo Clinic, Rochester, Minnesota, USA

BENJAMIN G. DOMB, MD
Founder and Medical Director, American Hip Institute, Chicago, Illinois, USA; Chair, American Hip Institute Research Foundation, Des Plaines, Illinois, USA

DAVID GE, MD
Fellow, Department of Orthopedic Surgery, Duke University Medical Center, Durham, North Carolina, USA

NICHOLAS GIRARDI, MD
Resident, Department of Orthopedic Surgery, The University of Texas at Austin Dell Medical School, Austin, Texas, USA

JOSHUA D. HARRIS, MD
Associate Professor, Department of Orthopaedics and Sports Medicine, Houston Methodist Hospital, Houston, Texas, USA; Associate Professor of Orthopaedic Surgery, Weill Cornell Medical College, New York, New York, USA

MARIO HEVESI, MD, PhD
Associate Professor of Orthopedic Surgery, Department of Orthopedic Surgery and Sports Medicine, Mayo Clinic, Rochester, Minnesota, USA

JASON G. INA, MD
Surgeon, Department of Orthopaedic Surgery, University Hospitals Drusinsky Sports Medicine Institute, Rainbow Babies and Children, University Hospitals, Cleveland, Ohio, USA

ADY H. KAHANA-ROJKIND, MD
Orthopedic Surgeon, Hip Preservation and Reconstruction Specialist, American Hip Institute Research Foundation, Chicago, Illinois, USA; Orthopedic Surgeon, Department of Orthopaedic Surgery, ABC Medical Center, Ortomove, Mexico City, Mexico

JOHN J. KELLY, MD
Fellow, Department of Orthopedic Surgery and Sports Medicine, Mayo Clinic, Rochester, Minnesota, USA

VIKAS KHANDUJA, MA (Cantab), MB BS, MSc, FRCS (TR & Orth), PhD
Hunterian Professor 2021, Royal College of Surgeons of England, Professor, Consultant Trauma and Orthopaedic Surgeon, Department of Trauma and Orthopaedic Surgery, Addenbrookes –Cambridge University Hospitals NHS Foundation Trust, Cambridge, United Kingdom

JOHN M. KOPRIVA, MD
Surgeon, Department of Orthopaedic Surgery, University Hospitals Drusinsky Sports Medicine Institute, Cleveland, Ohio, USA

AARON J. KRYCH, MD
Chair, Department of Orthopedic Surgery and Sports Medicine, Mayo Clinic, Rochester, Minnesota, USA

JESSICA LEE, MD
Assistant Professor, Department of Orthopedics, University of Colorado School of Medicine, Aurora, Colorado, USA

BRUCE A. LEVY, MD
Academic Chief of Sports Medicine, Director of Orthopedic Sports Medicine Fellowship, Department of Orthopedic Surgery, Orlando Health Jewett Orthopedic Institute, Orlando, Florida, USA

RICHARD C. MATHER III, MD, MBA
Assistant Professor, Vice Chairman, Practice Innovation, Department of Orthopedic Surgery, Duke University Medical Center, Durham, North Carolina, USA

OMER MEI-DAN, MD
Professor, Department of Orthopedics, University of Colorado School of Medicine, Aurora, Colorado, USA

TY L. MONTY, BSc
Research Assistants, Section of Young Adult Hip Surgery, Division of Sports Medicine, Department of Orthopedic Surgery, Rush University Medical Center, Chicago, Illinois, USA

SHANE J. NHO, MD, MS
Professor, Department of Orthopedic Surgery, Surgeon, Section of Young Adult Hip Surgery, Division of Sports Medicine, Midwest Orthopaedics at Rush, Rush University Medical Center, Chicago, Illinois, USA

ALEX R. OLES, MD, PhD
Resident, Department of Orthopedic Surgery and Sports Medicine, Mayo Clinic, Rochester, Minnesota, USA

ROGER QUESADA-JIMENEZ, MD
Orthopedic Surgeon, Hip Preservation and Reconstruction Specialist, American Hip Institute Research Foundation, Chicago, Illinois, USA

BRENDEN RONNA, MD
Fellow Physician, Department of Orthopedic Surgery, University of Wisconsin-Madison, Madison, Wisconsin, USA

MICHAEL J. SALATA, MD
Professor, Department of Orthopaedic Surgery, University Hospitals Drusinsky Sports Medicine Institute, Cleveland, Ohio, USA

JACOB J. SCHAEFER, MD
Resident Physician, Department of Orthopedic Surgery, Mayo Clinic, Rochester, Minnesota, USA

CHANDLER A. SPARKS, MSc, BSc
Research Assistants, Section of Young Adult Hip Surgery, Division of Sports Medicine, Department of Orthopedic Surgery, Rush University Medical Center, Chicago, Illinois, USA

LUKE S. SPENCER GARDNER, MD
Assistant Professor, Department of Orthopedic Surgery, Mayo Clinic, Jacksonville, Florida, USA

ANDREA SPIKER, MD
Assistant Professor, Department of Orthopedic Surgery, University of Wisconsin-Madison, Madison, Wisconsin, USA

Contents

CLINICS IN SPORTS MEDICINE

FORTHCOMING ISSUES

January 2027
Shoulder Arthritis
Matthew Deasey, *Editor*

April 2027
Imaging in Sports Medicine
Maxine Kresse and Michael Perry, *Editors*

July 2027
Spine Conditions and Injuries in the Athlete
Stephen Lockey, *Editor*

RECENT ISSUES

July 2026
Treatment Considerations of the Female Athlete
Emma L. Klosterman and Jonathan Goodloe, *Editors*

April 2026
Concussion and Head Injuries in Sports
Stephanie Alessi-LaRosa, *Editor*

January 2026
Osteotomies Around the Knee
Michael J. Alaia, *Editor*

SERIES OF RELATED INTEREST

Orthopedic Clinics
https://www.orthopedic.theclinics.com/
Foot and Ankle Clinics
https://www.foot.theclinics.com/
Hand Clinics
https://www.hand.theclinics.com/
Physical Medicine and Rehabilitation Clinics
https://www.pmr.theclinics.com/

Foreword

Intrepid Surgeon-Explorers: Mapping the New Frontiers of Hip Arthroscopy

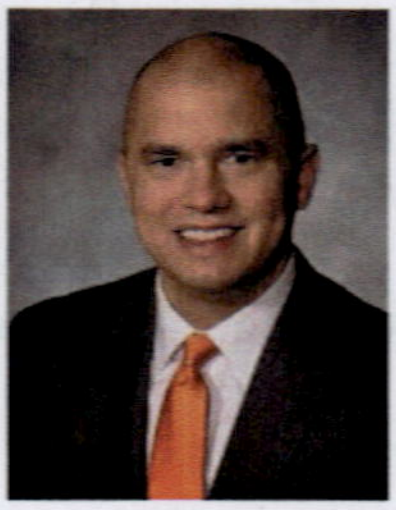

F. Winston Gwathmey, MD
Consulting Editor

In this issue of *Clinics in Sports Medicine*, guest editors Mario Hevesi and Shane Nho tackle a topic near and dear to my heart—hip arthroscopy. Eleven years ago, I was the guest editor of a *Clinics in Sports Medicine* issue entitled, "Hip Arthroscopy," in which we covered the fundamentals of this relatively new area of sports medicine. Fast forward a decade, and there has been extensive advancement in our collective understanding of hip pathology and a rapid progression in techniques. Surgeons have moved beyond the confines of the central compartment into new spaces around the hip. Like explorers, hip surgeons are venturing into uncharted territory and expanding the potential of hip arthroscopy.

This issue goes beyond the basics. Carefully selected experts introduce innovative approaches to access and portal placement, evolving strategies for labral management and reconstruction, advanced osteochondroplasty techniques, and capsular reconstruction. The role of arthroscopy in the management of hip dysplasia is reviewed. The mysteries of the posterior hip are explored in articles on ischiofemoral impingement and deep gluteal space. Importantly, the issue also addresses complications, emphasizing the principles of prevention, early recognition, effective management, and critical components of any evolving surgical field.

As hip arthroscopy continues to discover these new frontiers, the focus must remain on delivering durable, reproducible outcomes while preserving the native joint. This requires not only technical expertise but also sound judgment and an ongoing commitment to understanding the evolving evidence base. This issue provides a valuable framework for navigating these challenges and advancing the practice of hip preservation. We are not simply discovering new frontiers in hip arthroscopy, we are

Clin Sports Med 45 (2026) xiii–xiv
https://doi.org/10.1016/j.csm.2026.05.001
0278-5919/26/© 2026 Published by Elsevier Inc.

responsible for mapping them, defining their limits, and establishing the pathways that allow others to follow safely.

F. Winston Gwathmey, MD
Associate Professor of Orthopaedic Surgery
University of Virginia Health System
Charlottesville, Virginia, USA

Vice Chair for Orthopaedic Education
and Residency Program Director
Team Physician
UVA and JMU Athletics
Charlottesville, Virginia, USA

E-mail address:
FWG7D@uvahealth.org

Preface
To Sphericity and Beyond: New Frontiers in Hip Arthroscopy

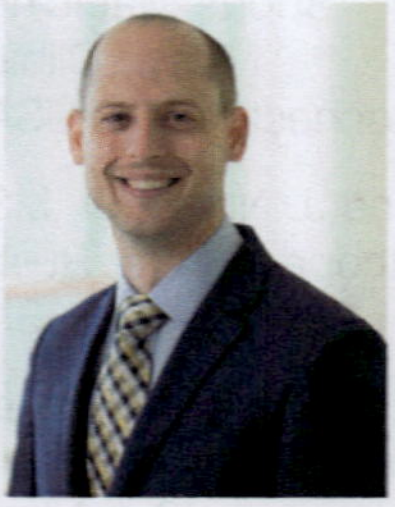
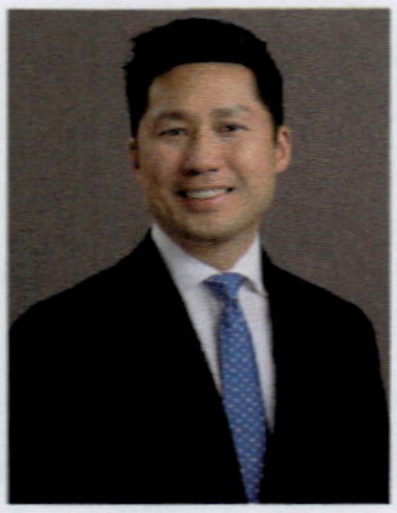

Mario Hevesi, MD, PhD Shane J. Nho, MD, MS
Editors

Hip arthroscopy continues to rapidly advance, with increasing attention turned to innovative techniques for percutaneous access, restoration and reconstruction of the labral suction seal, growing consideration of concomitant dysplasia treatment including osteotomy, capsular preservation, and also new frontiers into the peritrochanteric and gluteal space.

This issue focuses on novel additions to the toolbox of arthroscopic and endoscopic hip surgery. The topics presented are important as we shift to increasingly comprehensive, minimally invasive treatment of hip disorders ranging from impingement to dysplasia, ischiofemoral offset, and beyond. Readers will benefit from expert commentary and techniques in evolving areas of minimally invasive hip preservation surgery, while also gaining pearls and pitfalls to assist in the prevention, detection, and avoidance of complications in this ever-evolving field.

Join us, as we explore the new frontiers of hip arthroscopy.

DISCLOSURES

M. Hevesi discloses serving as consultant for Moximed, Stryker, and DJO, LLC; receiving IP Royalties from Elsevier; and serving on the editorial or governing board for *Journal of Cartilage and Joint Preservation.* S.J. Nho discloses serving as a board or committee member for American Orthopaedic Society for Sports Medicine and Arthroscopy Association of North America; receiving IP royalties from Ossur and

Clin Sports Med 45 (2026) xv–xvi
https://doi.org/10.1016/j.csm.2026.04.004
0278-5919/26/© 2026 Published by Elsevier Inc.

Stryker; receiving publishing royalties, financial or material support from Springer; and serving as a paid consultant for, and receiving research support from, Stryker.

Mario Hevesi, MD, PhD
Department of Orthopedic Surgery and
Sports Medicine
Mayo Clinic
Rochester, MN, USA

Shane J. Nho, MD, MS
Midwest Orthopaedics at Rush
Chicago, IL, USA

E-mail addresses:
hevesimario@gmail.com (M. Hevesi)
shane.nho@rushortho.com (S.J. Nho)

Percutaneous (Periportal) Hip Arthroscopy

Kristen I. Barton, MD, PhD, FRCSC, Ty L. Monty, BSc,
Chandler A. Sparks, MSc, BSc, Shane J. Nho, MD, MS*

KEYWORDS

- Arthroscopy • Hip arthroscopy • FAIS • Hip preservation • Capsulotomy
- Periportal • Periportal capsulotomy

KEY POINTS

- During hip arthroscopy, a capsulotomy is performed in order to achieve adequate visualization and working space for the instruments.
- Commonly used capsulotomy techniques, including the interportal capsulotomy and T-type capsulotomy, damage the iliofemoral ligament, an important anatomic structure for stability of the hip.
- Periportal capsulotomy is a relatively novel capsuloligamentous-preserving capsulotomy technique whereby 2 to 3 portals are created and then dilated.
- Current evidence supports improved patient outcomes from the periportal technique in hip arthroscopy for femoroacetabular impingement syndrome.

INTRODUCTION

Adequate visualization and working space within the hip joint are imperative for a successful hip arthroscopy. During hip arthroscopy, a capsulotomy is performed, whereby the fibrous joint capsule is incised, to achieve adequate visualization and access to both the central and peripheral compartments. However, failure to achieve proper capsular management during hip arthroscopy is recognized as a cause of pain, dysfunction, and reoperation.[1,2] Specifically, capsular insufficiency has been reported to account for up to 35% of revision cases.[1] Since that publication in 2007, there has been an abundance of literature focusing on capsular management in hip arthroscopy.[3–5]

Section of Young Adult Hip Surgery, Division of Sports Medicine, Department of Orthopedic Surgery, Rush University Medical Center, Chicago, IL, USA
* Corresponding author. Section of Young Adult Hip Surgery, Division of Sports Medicine, Department of Orthopedic Surgery, Rush University Medical Center, 1611 W. Harrison Street, Suite 300, Chicago, IL 60612.
E-mail address: shane.nho@rushortho.com

Clin Sports Med 45 (2026) 599–609
https://doi.org/10.1016/j.csm.2026.02.001 sportsmed.theclinics.com

Abbreviations	
ALP	anterolateral portal
DALA	distal anterolateral accessory
MAP	midanterior portal
ROM	range of motion

Several different types of capsulotomy techniques (eg, interportal capsulotomy, T-type capsulotomy, periportal capsulotomy) have been described previously, and there is debate as to which is the optimal technique.[6,7] Interportal capsulotomy represents the most used technique, where the capsule is incised between an anterolateral portal (ALP) and a midanterior portal (MAP) (**Fig. 1**A).[8] The T-type capsulotomy represents another incision, similar to the interportal capsulotomy, and an additional perpendicular incision along the anterior femoral head-neck junction (**Fig. 1**B).[7,8] The longitudinal incision of the T-type capsulotomy provides additional access and visualization of the peripheral compartment.

Both the interportal capsulotomy and the T-type capsulotomy disrupt the iliofemoral ligament, with a previous cadaveric study demonstrating that interportal capsulotomy results in violation of up to 74.2% of the width of the iliofemoral ligament.[9,10] The iliofemoral ligament, also referred to as the Y ligament, is the strongest ligament of the human body.[11] It arises from the anterior inferior iliac spine and acetabular rim, and then attaches to the intertrochanteric line.[12] The transverse, or lateral, band of the iliofemoral ligament is parallel to the axis of the femoral neck. In contrast, the descending, or medial, band runs parallel to the femoral shaft. Both bands play a major role in hip joint stability.[13]

In cadaveric studies, it has been shown that less force is required to distract the hip following interportal capsulotomy, with this effect being more pronounced with larger capsulotomy sizes.[14] Furthermore, hip macro-instability (ie, subluxation, dislocation) is known to occur in the setting of unrepaired capsulotomy owing to the inability of the capsule to resist anterior instability when the hip is extended and externally rotated.[15] Subtle instability, or micro-instability, is also recognized as a source of pain and degenerative changes that can result from hip arthroscopy capsulotomy.[16,17] Previous literature also has demonstrated that there are improved patient-reported

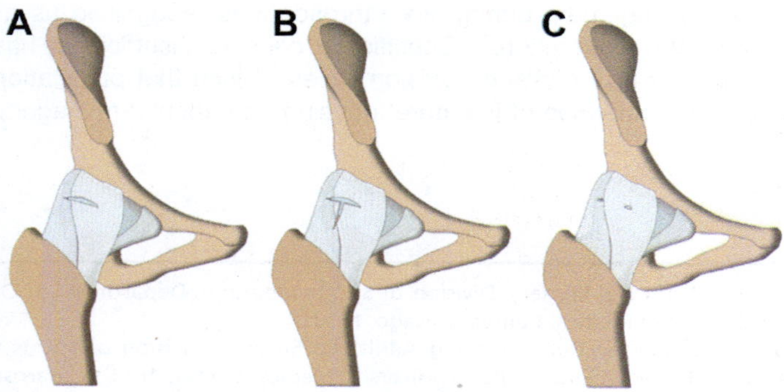

Fig. 1. Hip arthroscopy capsulotomy variations. (*A*) The interportal capsulotomy is carried out by incising the capsule between the ALP and MAP. (*B*) The T-type capsulotomy is achieved by extending an additional incision perpendicular to the interportal capsulotomy. (*C*) The periportal capsulotomy involves creating 2 punctures in the capsule that are dilated to 8 to 10 mm.

outcomes when the capsule is repaired, likely in part owing to the strength recovered in the iliofemoral ligament with capsular repair.[14,18] These studies draw attention to the importance of the iliofemoral ligament, and to the consequences of violation of the ligament.

To minimize impairment to the capsule during hip arthroscopy, relatively novel capsulotomy techniques have been described. One of these techniques is periportal capsulotomy, which uses 2 to 3 portals to gain access to the capsule (**Fig. 1**C).[19] Although technically challenging, the periportal capsulotomy has the advantage of limiting damage to the iliofemoral ligament and, therefore, possibly preventing iatrogenic hip instability.

The purpose of this article is to describe, in detail, the periportal surgical technique and its associated technical pearls. Furthermore, this article describes the current body of evidence surrounding the periportal capsulotomy, its advantages, disadvantages, and alternatives.

SURGICAL TECHNIQUE

Patient Positioning

A standard hip arthroscopy setup is required when attempting this percutaneous periportal capsulotomy. Briefly, the patient is placed supine on a traction table with their bilateral lower extremities placed securely in positioning boots to provide distraction. A large perineal post with padding is placed in an offset fashion, resting against the medial aspect of the nonoperative thigh. In periportal hip arthroscopy, gentle traction of the nonoperative limb is applied for stabilization of the patient perioperatively, while the operative limb is placed in a neutral position. Traction of the operative limb will be left down until assessment of the central compartment is ready to begin.

Peripheral Compartment

Standard hip arthroscopy normally begins with a central compartment approach where intraarticular pathologic condition is addressed. Subsequently, exploration of the peripheral compartment follows where extraarticular pathologic condition is treated. However, the converse has been described with periportal approaches.[20] Accessing and addressing the peripheral compartment first, then addressing the central compartment may allow for safer capsular management owing to decreased iatrogenic damage with fewer incisions made while also decreasing the time under tension of the distracted hip joint during the femoroplasty.[20] Furthermore, the decreased tension on the surrounding soft tissues allows for a greater "ballooning effect."

When using the percutaneous technique, portal selection and application are paramount for maintaining capsular integrity. Peripheral compartment approaches have been reported with an ALP, as this portal lies within the arthroscopy "safe zone."[21] Supplementary portal selection should be decided on based on preoperative planning and supposed intervention. Mindfulness of portal location can also dictate potential capsular management following the procedure. Specifically, the Mid-Anterior Portal (MAP) can damage the iliofemoral ligament and, although hip instability has been associated with the MAP portal using interportal capsulotomy and not periportal capsulotomy, caution should be exercised. Careful consideration with preoperative planning is advised. The percutaneous approach requires being comfortable with operating in a limited workspace. The surgeon should be nuanced in all perioperative movements while being mindful of preserving as much capsular integrity as possible.

With the hip in distraction, this technique begins by first creating the Mid-Anterior Portal (MAP) under fluoroscopy guidance using a spinal needle to briefly access the central

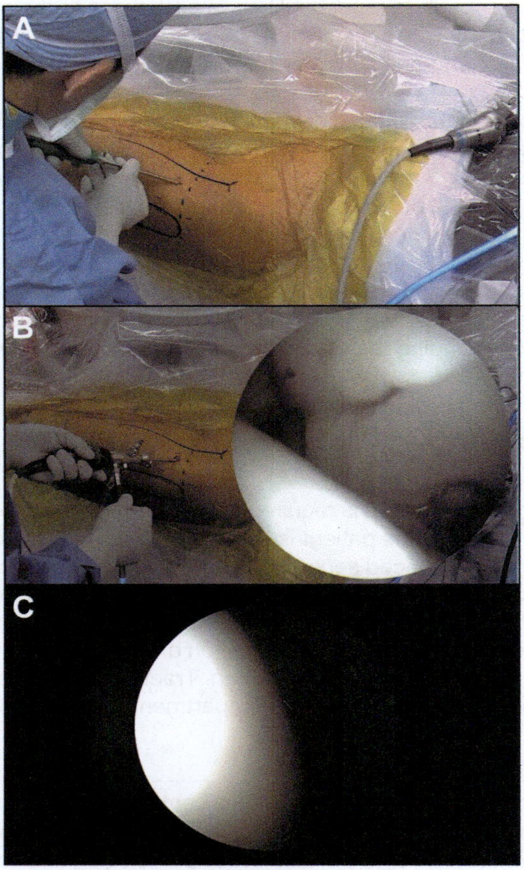

Fig. 2. MAP creation and diagnostic arthroscopy. (*A*) A spinal needle is used to establish entry into the capsule, minimizing iatrogenic damage to the capsule, followed by placement of a trocar. (*B*) A cannula is then placed into the central compartment. With the periportal approach, the cannula provides minimal dilation to the portals to allow increased accessibility. (*C*) With the hip off traction, the arthroscope is in the MAP, and saline can provide insufflation of the peripheral compartment.

compartment (**Fig. 2**A). Once the central compartment is easily visualized, a diagnostic arthroscopy of the central compartment is performed (**Fig. 2**B). The hip is taken off traction. The hip should be placed into 30° to 45° of flexion to relax the anterior capsule and allow for adequate insufflation of the compartment. A 70° arthroscope is installed into the MAP for evaluation of the peripheral compartment. Saline is then run through this space to increase visualization via the ballooning effect (**Fig. 2**C). Because of the limited capsulotomy, the inserted arthroscopy fluid does not seamlessly exit the peripheral compartment and thus expands the hip capsule more than what may be seen with a more intrusive capsulotomy approach. The pressure of the saline infusion causes the surrounding soft tissue to expand and not only improve visualization but also increase the available area for the surgeon to work in. With an increased workspace and improved visualization, addressing the femoral head/neck junction and other extraarticular pathologic condition becomes slightly less challenging.

Next, the anterolateral portal (ALP) is created under direct arthroscopic visualization with a spinal needle, nitinol wire, and 5.5-mm metal cannula to prepare for femoroplasty (**Fig. 3**A). Once the trocar has been established, a switching stick is placed into the metal canula. The 5.5-mm arthroscopic burr is taken apart on the back table, and the outer tube can be placed over the switching stick. The inner tube of the burr is placed

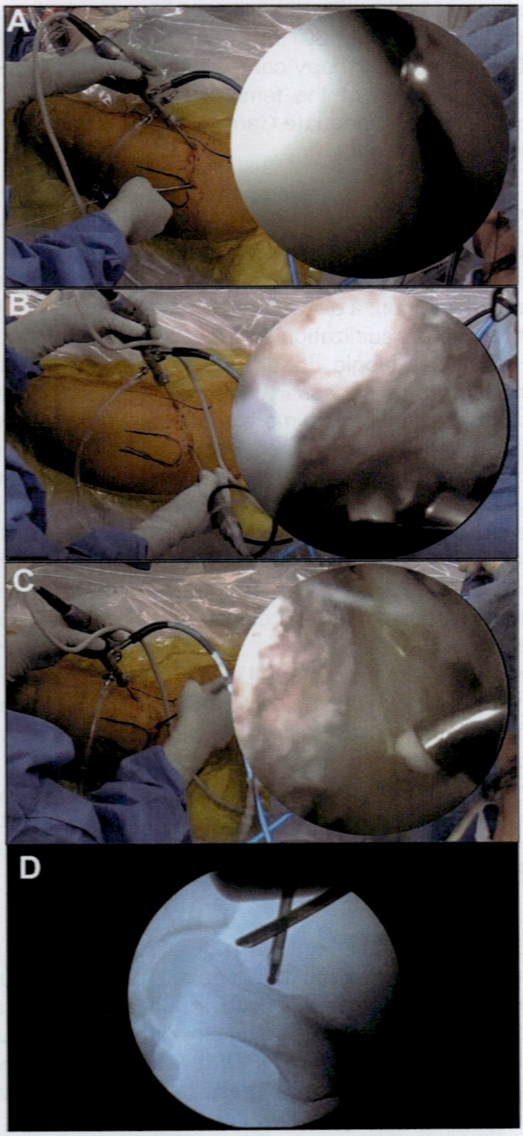

Fig. 3. Intraoperative arthroscopic view of the peripheral compartment following periportal capsulotomy. (*A*) Establishing the ALP using a trocar. (*B*) An arthroscopic burr can be inserted to perform osteochondroplasty of the Cam deformity. (*C*) A radiofrequency ablator can be used to remove periosteal tissue from the Cam deformity to allow for visualization of the proximal femur. (*D*) Femoral osteochondroplasty is carried out under fluoroscopic guidance.

in the outer tube, and then the rest of the instrument is attached to prevent further damage to the capsule. Osseous abnormalities are then addressed by femoroplasty of the causative CAM lesion under fluoroscopic guidance (**Fig. 3**B). In addition, a 4.0-mm arthroscopic shaver/radiofrequency ablator is used to address the periosteum or soft tissue following the femoroplasty (**Fig. 3**C). A dynamic hip examination is crucial to fully observe the femoral head and neck in its entirety under fluoroscopy and to ensure adequate Cam lesion correction. The assessment consists of evaluating the neck with 90° of flexion, approximately 30° of internal and external rotation, and then repeated at 60° of flexion. Fluoroscopy can be used throughout the femoroplasty to ensure that accurate resection of the femoral head and neck offset is achieved (**Fig. 3**D). Upon completing an adequate Cam decompression, attention can then be turned to the central compartment.

Central Compartment

The arthroscope is then shuttled from the MAP to the ALP for better visualization of the central compartment. The joint is then distracted to properly address any intraarticular pathologic condition. In addition, a distal anterolateral accessory (DALA) portal can be created under arthroscopic visualization to allow for appropriate anchor placement when addressing labral pathologic condition (**Fig. 4**A). An arthroscopic shaver is used to debride the labrum as necessary. The rim is then prepared with an arthroscopic burr by decortication to create a more accepting landing zone for labral sutures and promote reapproximation. Debridement of degenerative tissue of the labrum may be also performed, as necessary. Using the DALA portal, a straight wire drill guide will be used for placement of 1.4-mm polyetheretherketone suture anchors into the acetabulum for anatomic approximation of the torn labrum. Next, the arthroscope is placed into the MAP portal, and another anchor is placed through the ALP (**Fig. 4**B). Placement of sutures will occur every 8 to 10 mm along the tear to ensure proper fixation, ensuring that the least amount of foreign material as possible interfaces with the joint space (**Fig. 4**C).[21]

Following an adequate intraarticular labral repair, attention is then turned to managing the capsule. The arthroscope can be switched to the DALA for improved visualization of the plication in some cases. Although with periportal approaches, capsular damage is limited, it is still in the authors' practice to plicate the capsule and add further stability where able. Ultra-high-molecular-weight polyethylene sutures are used with standard arthroscopic techniques to complete the capsular plication (**Fig. 5**). A sufficient repair of the anterior hip capsule should be made to ensure capsular integrity.[22]

Postoperative Rehabilitation Protocol

Gradual progression of weight-bearing status occurs postoperatively. For the initial 1 to 2 weeks, flat foot partial weight-bearing with crutches or another assistive device is allowed. Weeks 3 to 6 can then be focused on slow increased ambulation and weight bearing as tolerated. Range of motion (ROM), specifically external rotation and abduction, are to be limited exclusively. These movements are to be restricted by the patient's hip brace throughout the first 6 weeks while working closely with their physical therapist about 2 times per week. After the conclusion of the 6-week mark, the patient can begin to progress in their strength training with their physical therapist. If tolerated, the weight-bearing restrictions can also be modified, and slow progression back to normal ROM can occur. Gait training at this point is also advised. At about 12 weeks postoperatively, the patient can begin to transition

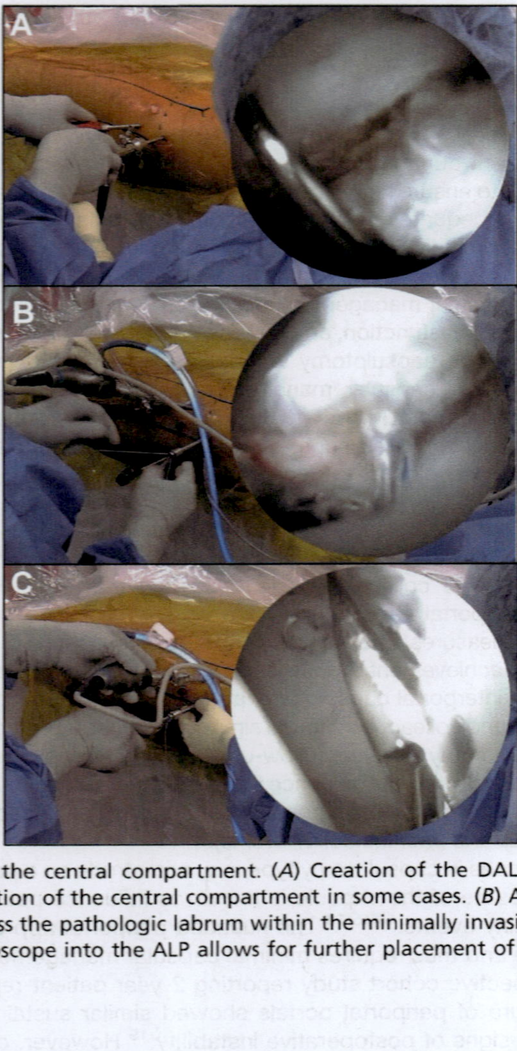

Fig. 4. Addressing the central compartment. (*A*) Creation of the DALA portal allows for improved visualization of the central compartment in some cases. (*B*) A drill guide and suture grasper address the pathologic labrum within the minimally invasive portal. (*C*) Placement of the arthroscope into the ALP allows for further placement of anchors for labrum repair.

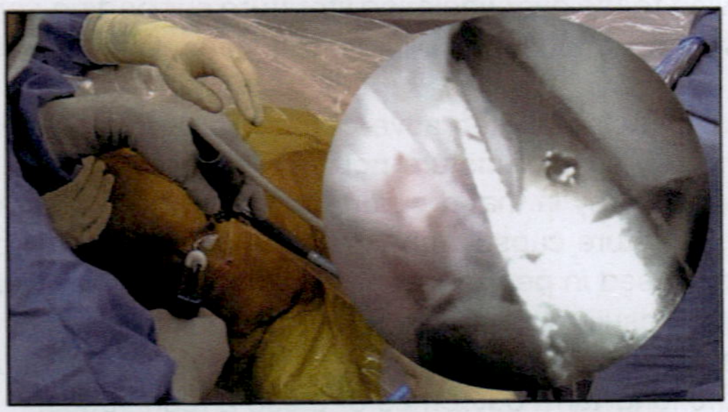

Fig. 5. Capsular plication with the arthroscope placed in the MAP and placement of ultra-high-molecular-weight polyethylene suture through the DALA.

back to normal activities, while after the 16-week mark, they can plan to return to sporting activities as tolerated.

DISCUSSION

Capsular management during hip arthroscopy is critical for restoring biomechanical properties of the hip to ensure high survivorship and an improvement in functional outcomes.[5] Despite an adequate repair and meticulous capsular management during hip arthroscopy, previous studies have demonstrated subluxation and dislocation events, microinstability, capsular irregularities, and heterotrophic ossification.[15,23,24] Failure to achieve adequate capsular management, including proper capsular integrity and tension, is a cause of pain, dysfunction, and revision surgery.[1,2,22] Although the interportal capsulotomy and T-type capsulotomy techniques in hip arthroscopy are the most common techniques for capsular management in hip preservation surgery, both methods violate the iliofemoral ligament. Although both are reproducible and safe procedures, further novel techniques, such as the periportal technique and puncture capsulotomy, have been developed to decrease the risk of capsular insufficiency and impairment.[25,26]

A handful of previous studies support the capsuloligamentous-preserving hip arthroscopy capsulotomy techniques, such as the periportal approach.[6,19,27] A recent systematic review by Klug and colleagues[28] demonstrated that patients undergoing hip arthroscopy with periportal capsulotomy showed improvements in multiple patient-reported outcome measures at a minimum of 2-year follow-up. McGovern and colleagues[27] found that achievement of patient-reported outcomes were similar irrespective of periportal versus interportal capsulotomy at a minimum of 2 years postoperatively. Similarly, Parvaresh and colleagues[29] found similar outcomes when comparing interportal and T-type capsulotomy at 2-year follow-up. These findings suggest in most routine cases, capsulotomy type may not influence the patient's prognosis but should be determined preoperatively based on the surgeon's comfort level and various patient factors (eg, joint laxity status and prior instability events).

Although differences in capsulotomy type may not intrude on a patient's prognosis in many cases, closure of the capsule is known to influence patient-reported outcomes and instability events.[14,15,18] The nuanced periportal approach creates less iatrogenic damage and thus requires minimal capsular management in most cases. A previous retrospective cohort study reporting 2-year patient-reported outcomes following nonclosure of periportal portals showed similar sustained improvement in patients and no signs of postoperative instability.[19] However, caution should be used in patients with previous joint laxity/instability and/or hip dysplasia. In the authors' practice, owing to the overwhelming literature supporting capsular closure improves outcomes, they choose to plicate the capsule even with the periportal approach.

Puncture capsulotomy is an alternative capsuloligamentous-preserving capsulotomy technique whereby small puncture portals are used.[30,31] This technique differs from periportal capsulotomy in that the portals are not dilated in puncture capsulotomy. Furthermore, puncture capsulotomy techniques often use 4 portals in contrast to the 2 to 3 typically used in periportal capsulotomy.[30,31] The current literature supports both puncture capsulotomy and periportal capsulotomy as effective techniques to access the capsule during hip arthroscopy.[28] However, there is currently limited evidence regarding the long-term outcomes of these 2 techniques.

With the periportal technique detailed here, there is limited tissue manipulation and damage to the capsule. The advantages of this method are the following: improves visualization and orientation, preserves anatomy (iliofemoral ligament and soft tissues), minimizes damage to the capsule, minimizes postoperative instability, minimizes the risk of heterotic ossification owing to minimally disturbing the soft tissues, and minimizes fluid extravasation.[6] The disadvantages of the periportal technique include the following: technical difficulty to perform and steep learning curve to perform and difficulty addressing peripheral compartment pathologic condition. Surgeons adapting this technique must be aware of these disadvantages and prioritize visualization and adequate management of the relevant pathologic condition, even at the expense of more extensive capsulotomy techniques (eg, interportal and T-type capsulotomy) if required.

Further investigation is warranted regarding long-term outcomes of the periportal capsulotomy technique and other related relatively novel capsuloligamentous-preserving capsulotomy techniques. Furthermore, studies comparing various capsulotomy techniques is warranted for a more robust understanding of how capsulotomy technique influences patient outcomes. Of particular interest regarding capsuloligamentous-preserving capsulotomy techniques is populations where innate instability may already be present. Two such patient populations include those with joint hypermobility (eg, Ehlers-Danlos syndrome) and borderline hip dysplasia. Future investigation is warranted to understand if capsuloligamentous-preserving capsulotomy techniques improve outcomes and decrease the incidence of instability in these groups. Last, there remains a need to better define the learning curve for these capsulotomy techniques and how outcomes may vary between high-volume and lower-volume settings given the technical difficulties of the technique.

SUMMARY

Commonly used capsulotomy techniques violate the iliofemoral ligament, which may introduce iatrogenic instability. Periportal capsulotomy is one technique to minimize impairment to the capsule during hip arthroscopy. Hip preservation surgeons should be aware of the advantages and disadvantages of the minimally invasive technique.

CLINICS CARE POINTS

- Capsulotomy during hip arthroscopy can result in instability to the hip joint if proper care is not taken to maintain capsular integrity.
- Periportal capsulotomy is a capsuloligamentous-preserving capsulotomy technique with promising patient-reported outcomes and reoperation-free survival.
- Introduction of instruments into the portals should be done with care to not introduce additional iatrogenic capsular damage and to maintain capsular pressure, which allows for the ballooning effect to aid in visualization.
- The 80-20 rule should be followed when introducing cannulas or dilators.[20] Following this rule, 80% of the motion should be twisting and 20% should be pushing. This minimizes the risk of cartilage or labral damage during introduction of cannulas or dilators to the portals.
- Using a sleeve of the shaver or burr as a cannula while switching between instrumentation during femoroplasty may help with joint entry.
- Proper portal placement is crucial to a successful hip arthroscopy procedure using this technique. Placement of the MAP too medially can limit lateral visualization of the head-neck junction, whereas placement too proximally may increase the risk of damage to the femoral head cartilage.

DISCLOSURES

K.I. Barton: BD Health: Consultant; American Academy of Hip and Knee Surgeons: Research committee member. S.J. Nho: American Orthopaedic Society for Sports Medicine: Board or committee member; Arthroscopy Association of North America: Board or committee member; Ossur: IP royalties; Springer: Publishing royalties, financial or material support; Stryker: IP royalties, paid consultant, research support.

REFERENCES

1. Philippon MJ, Schenker ML, Briggs KK, et al. Revision hip arthroscopy. Am J Sports Med 2007;35(11):1918–21.
2. Mortensen AJ, Metz AK, Froerer DL, et al. Hip capsular deficiency—a cause of post-surgical instability in the revision setting following hip arthroscopy for femoroacetabular impingement. Curr Rev Musculoskelet Med 2021;14(6):351–60.
3. Dasari SP, Kasson LB, Condon JJ, et al. Systematic review and meta-analysis of studies comparing complete capsular closure against unrepaired hip capsules during hip arthroscopy. Orthop J Sports Med 2023;11(10). https://doi.org/10.1177/23259671231197435.
4. Kunze KN, Vadhera A, Devinney A, et al. Effect of capsular closure after hip arthroscopy for femoroacetabular impingement syndrome on achieving clinically meaningful outcomes: a meta-analysis of prospective and comparative studies. Orthop J Sports Med 2021;9(6). https://doi.org/10.1177/23259671211017467.
5. Nho SJ, Beck EC, Kunze KN, et al. Contemporary management of the hip capsule during arthroscopic hip preservation surgery. Curr Rev Musculoskelet Med 2019;12(3):260–70.
6. Monroe EJ, Chambers CC, Zhang AL. Periportal capsulotomy: a technique for limited violation of the hip capsule during arthroscopy for femoroacetabular impingement. Arthrosc Tech 2019;8(2):e205–8.
7. Lee DR, Simon KN, Levy BA, et al. Capsular management in hip arthroscopy: interportal and t-capsulotomy, suspension, and closure. Arthrosc Tech 2024 13(3): 102893. https://doi.org/10.1016/j.eats.2023.102893.
8. Kerzner B, Dasari SP, Khan ZA, et al. Capsular management at the time of hip arthroscopy for femoroacetabular impingement syndrome varies with geography and surgeon subspecialty training: a cross-sectional, multinational surgeon survey. Arthrosc J Arthrosc Relat Surg 2024;40(11):2695–703.e1.
9. Cvetanovich GL, Levy DM, Beck EC, et al. A T-capsulotomy provides increased hip joint visualization compared with an extended interportal capsulotomy. J Hip Preserv Surg 2019;6(2):157–63.
10. Weber AE, Alluri RK, Makhni EC, et al. Anatomic evaluation of the interportal capsulotomy made with the modified anterior portal versus standard anterior portal: comparable utility with decreased capsule morbidity. Hip Pelvis 2020;32(1):42–9.
11. St-Pierre M, Effatparvar MR, Begon M, et al. Differentiation of strains in the lateral and medial bands of the iliofemoral ligament: a segmental approach. J Anat 2023;243(4):674–83.
12. Tsutsumi M, Nimura A, Akita K. New insight into the iliofemoral ligament based on the anatomical study of the hip joint capsule. J Anat 2020;236(5):946–53.
13. Martin HD, Savage A, Braly BA, et al. The function of the hip capsular ligaments: a quantitative report. Arthrosc J Arthrosc Relat Surg 2008;24(2):188–95.
14. Khair MM, Grzybowski JS, Kuhns BD, et al. The effect of capsulotomy and capsular repair on hip distraction: a cadaveric investigation. Arthrosc J Arthrosc Relat Surg 2017;33(3):559–65.

15. Duplantier NL, McCulloch PC, Nho SJ, et al. Hip dislocation or subluxation after hip arthroscopy: a systematic review. Arthrosc J Arthrosc Relat Surg 2016;32(7): 1428–34.
16. Dangin A, Tardy N, Wettstein M, et al. Microinstability of the hip: a review. Orthop Traumatol Surg Res 2016;102(8S):S301–9.
17. Kalisvaart MM, Safran MR. Microinstability of the hip–it does exist: etiology, diagnosis and treatment. J Hip Preserv Surg 2015;2(2):123–35.
18. Owens JS, Jimenez AE, Shapira J, et al. Capsular repair may improve outcomes in patients undergoing hip arthroscopy for femoroacetabular impingement: a systematic review of comparative outcome studies. Arthrosc J Arthrosc Relat Surg 2021;37(9):2975–90.
19. Chambers CC, Monroe EJ, Flores SE, et al. Periportal capsulotomy: technique and outcomes for a limited capsulotomy during hip arthroscopy. Arthrosc J Arthrosc Relat Surg 2019;35(4):1120–7.
20. Floyd ER, Kippes TL, Hardie KA, et al. A technique for peripheral compartment first and periportal access for hip arthroscopy. Arthrosc Tech 2025;14(2):103192. https://doi.org/10.1016/j.eats.2024.103192.
21. Byrd JWT, Pappas JN, Pedley MJ. Hip arthroscopy: an anatomic study of portal placement and relationship to the extra-articular structures. Arthrosc J Arthrosc Relat Surg 1995;11(4):418–23.
22. Domb BG, Philippon MJ, Giordano BD. Arthroscopic capsulotomy, capsular repair, and capsular plication of the hip: relation to atraumatic instability. Arthroscopy 2013;29(1):162–73.
23. Shu B, Safran MR. Hip instability: anatomic and clinical considerations of traumatic and atraumatic instability. Clin Sports Med 2011;30(2):349–67.
24. McCormick F, Slikker W, Harris JD, et al. Evidence of capsular defect following hip arthroscopy. Knee Surg Sports Traumatol Arthrosc 2014;22(4):902–5.
25. Byrd JWT. Avoiding the labrum in hip arthroscopy. Arthrosc J Arthrosc Relat Surg 2000;16(7):770–3.
26. Kelly BT, Weiland DE, Schenker ML, et al. Arthroscopic labral repair in the hip: surgical technique and review of the literature. Arthrosc J Arthrosc Relat Surg 2005;21(12):1496–504.
27. McGovern RP, Bucci G, Nickel BA, et al. Arthroscopic capsular management of the hip: a comparison of indications for and clinical outcomes of periportal versus interportal capsulotomy. Arthroscopy 2021;37(1):86–94.
28. Klug T, Fox JD, Rosa R, et al. Patients undergoing hip arthroscopy with periportal and puncture capsulotomy demonstrate favorable outcomes at short-term follow-up: a systematic review. Arthroscopy 2025. https://doi.org/10.1016/j.arthro.2025.01.027.
29. Parvaresh K, Rasio JP, Martin RL, et al. Achievement of meaningful clinical outcomes is unaffected by capsulotomy type during arthroscopic treatment of femoroacetabular impingement syndrome: results from the multicenter arthroscopic study of the hip (MASH) study group. Am J Sports Med 2021;49(3):713–20.
30. Gillinov SM, Siddiq BS, Cherian NJ, et al. Puncture capsulotomy technique during hip arthroscopy. JBJS Essent Surg Tech 2024;14(2). https://doi.org/10.2106/JBJS.ST.23.00061.
31. Eberlin CT, Kucharik MP, Abraham PF, et al. Puncture capsulotomy technique for hip arthroscopy: midterm functional outcomes. Orthop J Sports Med 2023;11(1). https://doi.org/10.1177/23259671221144056.

Accessory Portals in Hip Arthroscopy

Zachary S. Aman, MD[a,*], David Ge, MD[a],
Richard C. Mather III, MD, MBA[b]

KEYWORDS

- Hip arthroscopy accessory portals • Distal anterolateral accessory portal (DALA)
- Proximal anterolateral acessory portal (PALA)
- Proximal midanterior portal (PMAP / dienst portal)

KEY POINTS

- Inconsistent nomenclature and overlapping definitions have hindered standardization, clarity in description, and application of accessory portals.
- Accessory portals improve visualization, instrumentation trajectory, anchor placement, and suture management, supporting both basic hip arthroscopy and advanced labral and capsular reconstructive procedures.
- The distal anterolateral accessory portal offers improved acetabular rim access and anchor trajectory while maintaining a favorable safety profile when established using defined anatomic landmarks.
- The proximal anterolateral and proximal midanterior portals may enhance peripheral compartment exposure and capsular management, facilitating accurate femoroplasty while minimizing capsular disruuption and iatrogenic injury.
- Posterolateral and double distal anterolateral portals expand access to posterior pathology and improve suture organization, enabling safe and efficient management of complex cases.

INTRODUCTION

Over 18 portals have been described in the literature[1,2] for arthroscopic access to the central and peripheral compartments of the hip (**Table 1**), many of which overlap in nomenclature or are reported modifications to historically standard portal locations. While basic hip arthroscopy procedures may only warrant 2 or 3 portals,[3] accessory portals may facilitate improved access, facile instrumentation, safe anchor placement,

[a] Department of Orthopedic Surgery, Duke University Medical Center, Durham, NC, USA; [b] Practice Innovation, Department of Orthopedic Surgery, Duke University Medical Center, Durham, NC, USA
* Corresponding author. Duke University School of Medicine, Department of Orthopedic Surgery, DUMC Box 104002, IPE - 311 Trent Drive, Durham, NC 27710.
E-mail address: zachary.aman@duke.edu

Clin Sports Med 45 (2026) 611–620
https://doi.org/10.1016/j.csm.2026.03.006 sportsmed.theclinics.com
0278-5919/26/

Abbreviations	
AL	anterolateral portal
ASIS	anterior superior iliac spine
DALA	distal anterolateral accessory portal
dDALA	double distal anterolateral accessory portal
LCFN	lateral femoral cutaneous nerve
MAP	midanterior portal
PALA	proximal anterolateral acessory portal
PL	posterolateral portal
PMAP	proximal midanterior portal

and suture management for a variety of procedures ranging from basic cam resection and labral repair, to more advanced complex procedures such as arthroscopic labral and capsular reconstruction. Descriptions of accessory portals for hip arthroscopy have historically been unclear in regards to naming and location, and review of the current literature finds that technique papers often refer to otherwise identical portal locations with unique nomenclature that coincide with advancements in surgical technique, further convoluting understanding and technical advancement in hip arthroscopy for the learning arthroscopist.[1] In this article, we will define common accessory portals and deconvolute historical nomenclature, and further describe their respective anatomic considerations and utility to address basic and complex pathology of the central and peripheral compartment.

Table 1
Summary of portals and associated references reported in the literature

Portal	References
AL	Robertson et al,[1] 2008; Thorey et al,[2] 2013, Chahla et al,[3] 2024
MAP	Robertson et al,[1] 2008; Degen et al,[4] 2017; Dumont et al,[5] 2019, Chahla et al,[3] 2024
DALA	Maldonado et al,[1] 2020; Thorey et al,[2] 2013; Degen et al,[4] 2017; Dumont et al,[5] 2019; Stanton et al,[1] 2016, Chahla et al,[3] 2024
dDALA	Senior author's preferred technique
Proximal AL Accessory Portal (PALA)	Christian et al,[6] 2023; Robertson et al,[1] 2008
PMAP/Dienst portal	Dienst et al,[7] 2005; Dantas et al,[8] 2020; Floyd et al,[9] 2025; Robertson et al,[1] 2008; Bhatia et al,[10] 2016
PL	Meta et al,[11] 2024; Robertson et al,[1] 2008; Chen et al,[12] 2023; Foster et al,[13] 2015; Zumstein et al,[14] 2009; Scott et al,[15] 2022; White et al,[16] 2020
Anterior Portal	Robertson et al,[1] 2008; Thorey et al,[2] 2013
Peritrochanteric space portal	Robertson et al,[1] 2008, Byrd et al,[17] 2013

This table aims to deconvolute previous descriptions and nomenclature when reviewing the primary literature.

ACCESSORY PORTALS FOR BASIC HIP ARTHROSCOPY

Distal Anterolateral Portal

The distal anterolateral accessory portal (DALA) is typically positioned 4 to 7 cm distal to the standard anterolateral (AL) portal along the femoral axis. Anatomically, the portal lies lateral to the greater trochanter and distal to the AL portal, which minimizes the risk to the lateral femoral cutaneous nerve (LCFN) and major vascular structures.[2,18] This trajectory provides improved access to the acetabular rim, particularly between the 2:30 and 9 o'clock positions, facilitating accurate and safe suture anchor placement. In addition, the DALA portal avoids hand crossover and suture entanglement during complex labral or capsular repairs due to the distal positioning of the portal. Compared with the midanterior portal (MAP), the DALA portal has a similar risk of intra-articular penetration and violation of the subchondral surface during anchor drilling.[4,5] Stanton and colleagues found in their cadaveric study that when using a straight drill guide, the DALA portal may decrease the incidence of intra-articular penetration compared to drilling through the AL or MAPs.[19] Patients who benefit most from the DALA portal include those with femoroacetabular impingement, labral tears, and chondral or capsular pathology requiring improved anchor trajectory or complex suture management.

Pearls for this technique include the use a spinal needle to establish the trajectory for the DALA portal starting about 3 to 4 cm distal to the AL portal in line with the femoral axis, fluoroscopy may help with the trajectory if necessary. With the camera viewing from the AL portal, the spinal needle should enter right through the subcutaneous tissue superficial to the capsule onto your intended position along the acetabular rim. Surgeons should take care placing anchors in the anterior and medial rim (2–4 o'clock positions) to prevent intra-articular and psoas tunnel perforation.

Pitfalls when using the DALA portal include portal placement medial to the anterior superior iliac spine (ASIS), risking damage to the LCFN—using anatomic landmarks is essential to stay lateral to the ASIS and distal to the AL portal. Furthermore, one should avoid overly distal portal placement, which may limit access to certain acetabular rim positions. Suture disorganization during complex capsular or labral reconstruction can lead to entanglement—consider using a double DALA (dDALA) technique in these advanced cases as described later in this article (**Fig. 1**A, B).

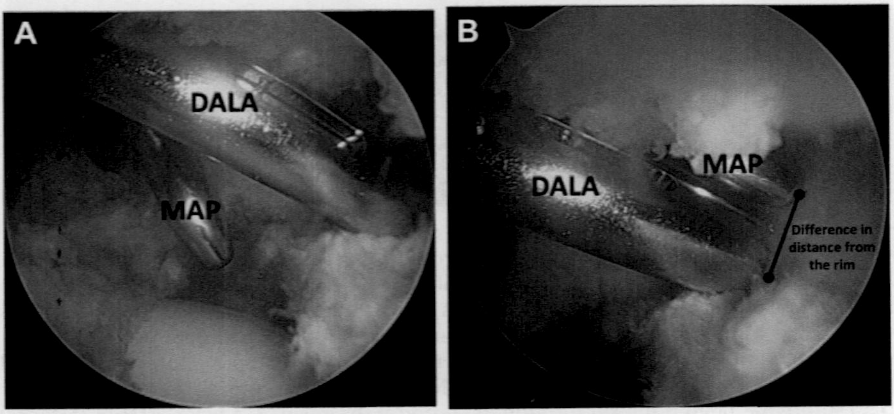

Fig. 1. This figure depicts the more advantageous trajectory for anchor placement for labral repair produced by the DALA portal. In (*A*), the difference in the angles between the MAP (switching stick in the cannula) and the DALA (drill guide) can be seen. (*B*) Shows how much closer to the rim the anchor placement can be with the DALA portal.

Proximal Anterolateral Acessory Portal

Capsular management with retention sutures and careful portal placement are critical to optimizing visualization of the peripheral compartment. The proximal AL portal (PALA), localized approximately 4 cm proximal to the AL portal along the same longitudinal axis,[1,6] serves to redirect the vector of traction on the capsule by rerouting capsular suspension sutures of T-capsulotomy leaflets.[6] This altered retraction vector shifts the capsular retraction posteriorly, markedly improving the arthroscopic field of view and enabling more complete and precise femoroplasty.[6] It should be noted that this portal location should not be confused with the proximal MAP (PMAP) or Dienst portal, which often is referred to as a PALA. This distinction will be further clarified in the next section of this article.

The PALA portal also offers several other advantages in addition to improved visualization. The traction vector also enhances capsular management by reducing mechanical stress on the capsular tissue, and retract the capsule away from the femoral neck decreasing iatrogenic damage risk while burring. Furthermore, the improved exposure afforded by the PALA portal can permit a shorter T-limb incision, thereby limiting unnecessary capsulotomy length while maintaining optimal visualization. During capsular closure, the redirected suture tension provides balanced resistance, allowing for efficient and precise suture passage, particularly with figure-of-8 configurations used to reapproximate the capsule. Collectively, these benefits improve both the accuracy of the osteoplasty and the quality of capsular repair. Despite its advantages, when used only for capsule suspension sutures, the PALA portal introduces a small additional incision and a brief increase in operative time. However, the portal is typically small—often requiring no formal closure at the capsular level.[6] (**Fig. 2**A, B).

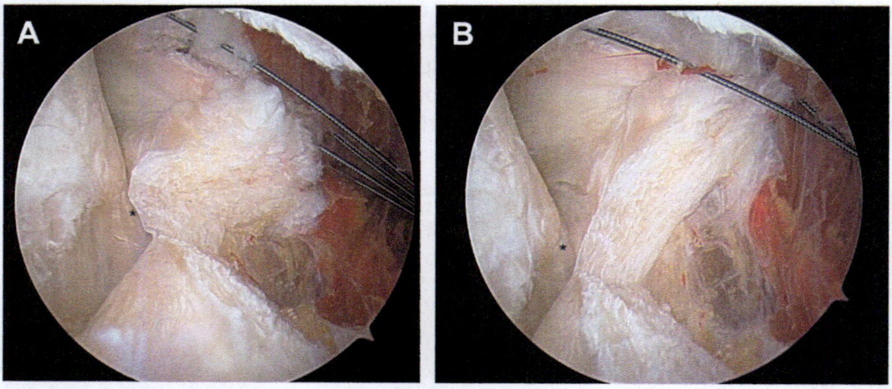

Fig. 2. (*A*) Arthroscopic photo of peripheral compartment exposure after T-capsulotomy with capsular retention sutures tensioned through AL and DALA portals. A black asterisk (*asterisk*) has been added overlying the lateral CAM lesion to highlight the capsular tissue obstructing view before redirection of sutures through the PALA portal. This photo shows how the line of pull through the AL portal can bunch this limb and does not consistently retract the capsule away from the femoral neck. (*B*) Arthroscopic photo of peripheral compartment exposure with capsular retention sutures after the distal lateral capsular (DLC) suture has been retrieved through PALA portal. As in **Fig. 2**, a black asterisk (*asterisk*) has been added overlying the lateral CAM lesion. In this figure, the asterisk highlights the improved visualization of the CAM lesion now that the capsular tissue is no longer obstructing due to the redirection of sutures through the PALA portal. It is also in a better position for capsule closure at the completion of the osteoplasty.

Proximal Midanterior Portal

Originally described by Dienst and colleagues, the PMAP or *Dienst* portal is located by palpating the soft spot found at one-third the distance along a line drawn from the ASIS to the tip of the greater trochanter. This portal location can also be found at the proximal vertex of the equilateral triangle formed between the AL portal and anterior portal. It is important to also note that this portal was originally referred to as the AL portal in 2005, and has also been cited in other technique papers as the PALA.[7–9] However, in this article we will uniformly refer to this portal location as the PMAP from here on, in accordance to how it was described by Robertson and colleagues (**Fig. 3**).

This portal was originally described as a viewing portal, allowing for safe access to the peripheral compartment aiming at the junction of the femoral head and neck, avoiding iatrogenic damage to the femoral cartilage, and popularized as a useful portal for *peripheral compartment first* access to the hip joint,[8,9] and other capsular sparing techniques for femoroacetabular impingement (FAI) pathology by avoiding transection of the iliofemoral ligament. This portal is relatively safe, and greater than 5 cm away from gluteal vessels and nerves. Several techniques have been described using the PMAP, and offers a useful working portal for instrument trajectory to address cam lesions, value in visualization of the peripheral compartment with the use of a capsular traction stitch through its innate retraction vector,[9] and also for 12 to 1 o'clock suture limb management for labral reconstruction as described by Bhatia and colleagues[10] Other advantages of the PMAP include easy accessibility and resection of anterosuperior pincer lesions and elevation of the anterosuperior labrum off the acetabular rim. The PMAP portal is also used for suture management in several techniques including capsule sparing techniques, labral reconstruction and occasionally capsule reconstruction (**Fig. 4**A, B).

A summary of basic arthroscopy portals and their location, technical application, and safety considerations can be found in **Table 2**.

HIP ARTHROSCOPY ACCESSORY PORTALS FOR ADVANCED HIP ARTHROSCOPY

Posterolateral Portal

The posterolateral portal (PL) remains a mainstay for addressing posteriorly based lesions of the hip, offering improved visualization of the posterior rim, labrum, and peripheral compartment, as well as optimized trajectory for instrumentation for posterior rim resection and labral repair.[11] However, a thorough understanding of the

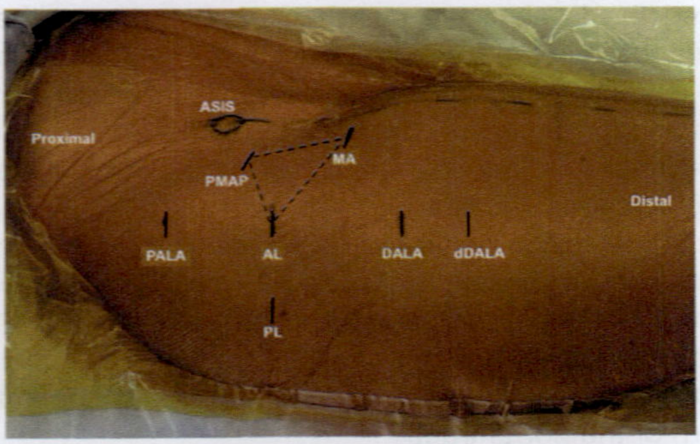

Fig. 3. Standard and accessory portals for arthroscopy of a right hip. *Abbreviation*: MA, midanterior.

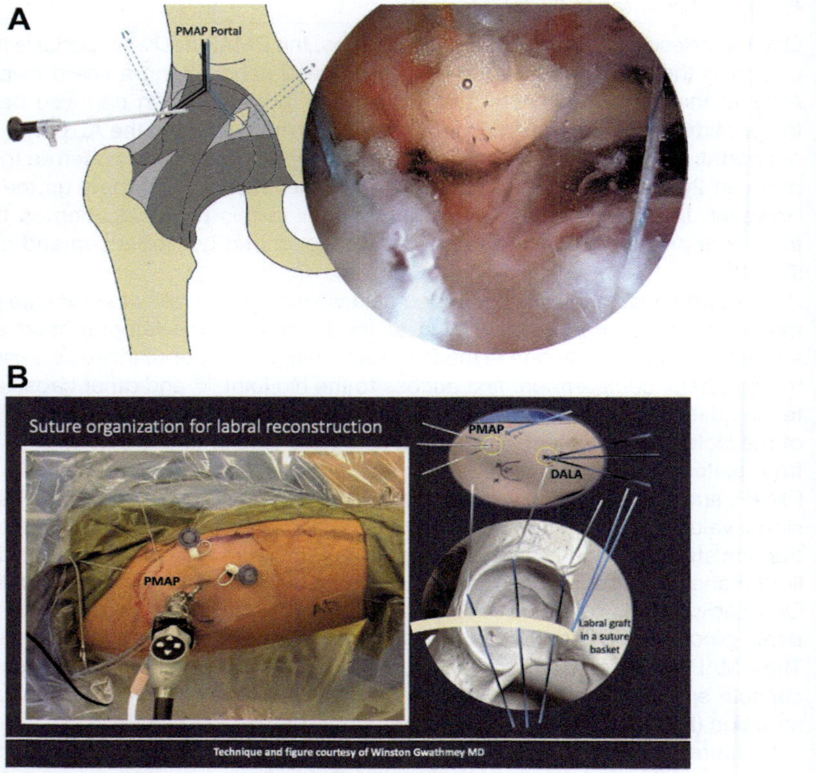

Fig. 4. (*A*) Shows the PMAP portal being used in a capsule sparing (periportal) approach to pull the 2 portal stitches in different directions to keep this portal open for more streamlined access to the joint. (*B*) Shows the PMAP portal being used for suture management in a labral reconstruction technique performed by Dr Winston Gwathmey MD. One set of sutures are pulled through the PMAP portal and the other through the DALA portal creating a basket that the graft is passed through. This effectively passes all sutures around the graft at once. (*Image Courtesy*: (b) Dr Winston Gwathmey MD.)

surrounding anatomy is essential for safe placement and instrumentation. Creation of the PL is typically made approximately 1 to 2 cm posterior to the tip of the greater trochanter matching the level of the standard AL portal, and the spinal needle is entered into the joint through the superior/lateral border of the ischiofemoral ligament, penetrating at the 10 o'clock position under direct visualization from the MAP.

Historic reservations for the use of the PL are related to the close proximity of the sciatic nerve, gluteal vessels, and the medial circumflex femoral artery and relative risk for injury. Robertson and colleagues reported that the average distance from the PL portal tract to the sciatic nerve is approximately 21 mm, although the minimal distance measured in cadavers was as close as 11 mm. Proximity of the sciatic nerve can also be dependent on hip flexion and rotation, and therefore it is important to be cognizant of patient positioning before portal creation and maintaining neutral hip position. Similarly, on average, terminal branches of the medial circumflex femoral artery may lie within 5 mm of the portal tract.

While the majority of labral tears occur between the 12 o'clock and 3 o'clock positions, labral tears and concomitant posterior rim pathology that extend posterior

Table 2
Summary of commonly used standard and accessory portals for basic hip arthroscopy, detailing anatomic location, technical applications, and key safety considerations

Portal	Description of Location	Technical Application	Safety Considerations
AL	Standard portal placed just anterior and superior to the tip of the greater trochanter	Primary viewing portal for central compartment access; used for diagnostic arthroscopy, interportal capsulotomy, and instrument triangulation	Established safe portal with predictable anatomy; care required to avoid cartilage scuffing during entry
Midanterior	Located approximately midway between the ASIS and the AL portal	Common working portal for labral work, suture passage, and peripheral compartment visualization	Increased proximity to the LFCN; careful localization required
DALA	Positioned 4–7 cm distal to the AL portal along the femoral axis, lateral to the greater trochanter	Optimizes acetabular rim access (2:30–9 o'clock), anchor trajectory, suture management, and avoidance of hand crossover; commonly used for labral and capsular repair	Must remain lateral to ASIS to avoid LFCN injury; anterior/medial anchor placement requires caution to prevent intra-articular or psoas tunnel perforation
PALA	Approximately 4 cm proximal to the AL portal along the same longitudinal axis as the AL and DALA portals	Redirects capsular suspension suture vectors during T-capsulotomy, improving peripheral compartment visualization, femoroplasty accuracy, and capsular closure	Minimal added morbidity; typically small and does not require capsular closure; adds minor operative time
PMAP/ Dienst portal	Located at the proximal vertex of an equilateral triangle formed by the AL and APs; ~one-third distance from ASIS to greater trochanter	Viewing or working portal for peripheral compartment–first access, cam resection, pincer correction, and labral reconstruction suture management	Generally safe with >5 cm clearance from major neurovascular structures

Abbreviation: MA, midanterior.

and lateral to the 12 o'clock position can be technically challenging to address through standard AL or MAPs due to suboptimal instrumentation trajectory. For posteriorly based labral tears, safe drilling and anchor placement can be instrumented through the PL while viewing through the MAP, with optimized trajectory to avoid violation of the articular cartilage and solid anchor fixation especially at the 8 o'clock to 10 o'clock positions.[12,13] Curved guides and the use of fluoroscopy can also be used to ensure safe placement. In these cases, the AL portal is then used for suture limb management. The PL also offers sufficient access to the posterior acetabular rim to address posterosuperior pincer lesions, and visualization of the posterior extent of anterosuperiorly based lesions. Zumstein and colleagues reported that posterosuperior pincer lesions may be underestimated without the addition of a PL, resulting in under resection.[14] The PL can also be valuable in protecting the posterior capsule during treatment of posterior acetabular pathology. Posterior capsule suspension sutures can be placed through the AL portal but the line of pull is typically oblique from the AL portal. This does not lift the capsule away from the rim to protect it and allow access. Retrieving those sutures through the PL creates a more perpendicular line of pull that substantially improves access and preserves the posterior capsule for repair. In complex cases such as larger labral reconstructions, the PL also allows for more facile triangulation and instrument maneuverability, which are critical for graft measurement, tensioning, and passage. This is especially useful in circumferential or posterior segment reconstructions are performed.[15,16]

Double Distal Anterolateral Accessory Portal

The dDALA is most often used in capsular reconstruction or revision cases to park the distal sutures to improve suture organization and efficiency. In this particular technique, a second DALA portal is created slightly distal or proximal to the first DALA portal.

A summary of advanced arthroscopy portals and their location, technical application, and safety considerations can be found in **Table 3**.

Table 3
Summary of commonly used standard and accessory portals for advanced hip arthroscopy, detailing anatomic location, technical applications, and key safety considerations

Portal	Description of Location	Technical Application	Safety Considerations
dDALA	Second portal created slightly proximal or distal to the primary DALA	Advanced suture organization and management during capsular or labral reconstruction and revision procedures	Additional incision; requires deliberate planning to avoid clutter and excessive portal crowding
Posterolateral	1–2 cm posterior to the tip of the greater trochanter at the level of the AL portal	Access to posterior acetabular rim, posterior labral tears (8–10 o'clock), posterior pincer lesions, and posterior capsular suspension	Close proximity to sciatic nerve and medial circumflex femoral artery; neutral hip positioning and careful trajectory essential

SUMMARY

This article serves to define accessory portal nomenclature and discusses several accessory portals that may be useful in facilitating improved peripheral and central compartment access, facile instrumentation, safe anchor placement, and advantages in facilitating suture and capsular management for hip arthroscopy. It is encouraged to recognize differences in portal nomenclature when applying accessory portals to standard clinical practice, and to continue to refer to these portals in a uniform manner when describing future arthroscopic techniques.

CLINICS CARE POINTS

- Precise portal localization using bony landmarks and spinal needle confirmation is essential to minimize neurovascular injury, particularly when establishing midanterior, distal anterolateral accessory portal (DALA), or posterolateral portals.
- The DALA portal improves anchor trajectory and suture management but should remain lateral to the anterior superior iliac spine to reduce the risk of lateral femoral cutaneous nerve injury.
- Redirecting capsular suspension sutures through proximal portals, such as the proximal anterolateral sportal, can substantially improve peripheral compartment visualization and reduce iatrogenic femoral neck injury during femoroplasty.
- Posterolateral portal use requires careful attention to hip position and trajectory, as proximity to the sciatic nerve and medial circumflex femoral artery increases risk with improper placement.
- In complex labral or capsular reconstruction, use of a second distal anterolateral portal may improve suture organization and efficiency but should be planned to avoid excessive portal crowding.

DISCLOSURE

Richard C. Mather III, MD, MBA, reports the following disclosures: AAOS: Board or committee member International Society of Hip Arthroscopy: Board or committee member North Carolina Orthopaedic Association: Board or committee member Pattern Health: Stock or stock Options. SCA Health: Employee. Springer: Publishing royalties, financial or material support. Stryker: IP royalties; Paid consultant, United Health Group: Stock or stock Options. Zachary Aman, MD, and David Ge, MD, have no disclosures.

REFERENCES

1. Robertson WJ, Kelly BT. The safe zone for hip arthroscopy: a cadaveric assessment of central, peripheral, and lateral compartment portal placement. Arthrosc J Arthrosc Relat Surg 2008;24(9):1019–26.
2. Thorey F, Ezechieli M, Ettinger M, et al. Access to the hip joint from standard arthroscopic portals: a cadaveric study. Arthrosc J Arthrosc Relat Surg 2013;29(8):1297–307.
3. Chahla J, Villarreal-Espinosa JB, Gonzalez Ayala S, et al. Basic hip arthroscopy part 1: patient positioning and portal placement. Arthrosc Tech 2024;13(12):103220.
4. Degen RM, Poultsides L, Mayer SW, et al. Safety of hip anchor insertion from the midanterior and distal anterolateral portals with a straight drill guide: a cadaveric study. Am J Sports Med 2017;45(3):627–35.

5. Dumont GD, Money AJ, Thier ZT. Acetabular subchondral and cortical perforation during labral repair with suture anchors: influence of portal location, curved versus straight drill guides, and drill starting point. Arthrosc J Arthrosc Relat Surg 2019;35(8):2349–54.
6. Christian RA, Cabell GH, Jarvis DL, et al. Proximal anterolateral accessory portal use improves peripheral compartment access and capsular management with T-Capsulotomy. Arthrosc Tech 2023;12(2):e161–5.
7. Dienst M, Seil R, Kohn DM. Safe arthroscopic access to the central compartment of the hip. Arthrosc J Arthrosc Relat Surg 2005;21(12):1510–4.
8. Dantas P, Gonçalves S, Mascarenhas V, et al. Hip arthroscopy with initial access to the peripheral compartment: a detailed step-by-step technique description. Arthrosc Tech 2020;9(11):e1651–5.
9. Floyd ER, Kippes TL, Hardie KA, et al. A technique for peripheral compartment first and periportal access for hip arthroscopy. Arthrosc Tech 2025;14(2):103192.
10. Bhatia S, Civitarese DM, Turnbull TL, et al. A novel repair method for radial tears of the medial meniscus: biomechanical comparison of transtibial 2-tunnel and double horizontal mattress suture techniques under cyclic loading. Am J Sports Med 2016;44(3):639–45.
11. Meta F, Rudisill SS, Simon KN, et al. Posterolateral acetabular labral repair: drilling using a percutaneous posterolateral portal. Arthrosc Tech 2024;13(7):102994.
12. Chen Q, Zou J, Wang F, et al. Portal selection for suture anchor placement during hip arthroscopic labral repair: a study based on 3-dimensional model reconstruction. Orthop J Sports Med 2023;11(8):23259671231189729.
13. Foster AD, Ryan J, Ellis T, et al. Safe suture anchor insertion for anterior and posterior hip labral repair. Journal of Hip Preservation Surgery 2015;2(2):170–4.
14. Zumstein M, Hahn F, Sukthankar A, et al. How accurately can the acetabular rim be trimmed in hip arthroscopy for pincer-type femoral acetabular impingement: a cadaveric investigation. Arthrosc J Arthrosc Relat Surg 2009;25(2):164–8.
15. Scott EJ. Editorial commentary: segmental hip labral reconstruction may be superior to circumferential reconstruction: bigger isn't better. Arthrosc J Arthrosc Relat Surg 2022;38(2):349–51.
16. White BJ. Editorial commentary: no longer a salvage procedure: allograft labral reconstruction of the hip rivals the results of labral repair. Arthrosc J Arthrosc Relat Surg 2020;36(10):2611–3.
17. Byrd JWT. Peritrochanteric access and gluteus medius repair. Arthrosc Tech 2013;2(3):e243–6.
18. Maldonado DR, Rosinsky PJ, Shapira J, et al. Stepwise safe access in hip arthroscopy in the supine position: tips and pearls from A to Z. J Am Acad Orthop Surg 2020;28(16):651–9.
19. Stanton M, Banffy M. Safe angle of anchor insertion for labral repair during hip arthroscopy. Arthrosc J Arthrosc Relat Surg 2016;32(9):1793–7.

Addressing the Everted Labrum: Advancement and Beyond

Nicholas Girardi, MD[a,*], Jessica Lee, MD[b], Omer Mei-Dan, MD[b]

KEYWORDS

• Everted labrum • Hip preservation • Hip arthroscopy • Labral advancement
• Labral reconstruction • Suction seal • Hip instability

KEY POINTS

- An everted acetabular labrum is a native pathologic labral variant.
- Diagnosis is made intraoperatively, seen as gapping between labrum and femoral head with the hip off traction.
- Restoration of the labral suction seal is the goal of surgical management.
- Treatment consists of labral advancement, augmentation, or reconstruction.
- Inside-out labral repair is the preferred technique due to the creation of force vectors that encourage restoration of the suction seal.

INTRODUCTION

The acetabular labrum is a fibrocartilaginous structure that acts as an extension of the bony acetabulum, playing a critical role in hip function and stability.[1–4] The acetabular labrum creates a suction seal over the femoral head.[1,3] Direct apposition of the labrum and femoral head generates pressurization of the joint with synovial fluid, which is thought to dissipate joint reactive forces and play a pivotal role in overall hip kinematics.[2]

Numerous anatomic acetabular labral variants have been described in the literature. Knowledge of these variants is important, as some commonly encountered variants are pathologic. The recently described native everted acetabular labrum is a pathologic labral variant, in which the acetabular labrum faces away from the femoral head.[5,6] This prevents apposition between the femoral head and labrum resulting in a dysfunctional labrum and compromise of the physiologic suction seal. These everted labra are commonly hypoplastic in size and assume a blunted or rounded shape on MRI.[5,6] The origin of the everted labrum is not fully understood; however, it has been hypothesized to be correlated with acetabular development starting from a tethered position leading to aberrant labral development. One theory, coined

[a] Department of Orthopedic Surgery, The University of Texas at Austin Dell Medical School, Austin, TX, USA; [b] Department of Orthopedics, University of Colorado School of Medicine
* Corresponding author. Department of Surgery and Perioperative Care, Dell Medical School, 1601 Trinity Street, Building B, Austin, TX 78712.
E-mail address: Nicholas.girardi@ascension.org

Clin Sports Med 45 (2026) 621–631
https://doi.org/10.1016/j.csm.2026.01.001 sportsmed.theclinics.com

Abbreviations	
FAI	femoracetabular impingement
PAO	periacetabular osteotomy

the growth mismatch theory, theorizes a difference in labral and acetabular rim growth during development, resulting in the labrum position being flipped to the capsular side of the rim. Over the course of development, once malpositioned on the capsular side of the acetabular rim, the labrum slowly stretches and slowly thins forming a symptomatic everted labrum.[6]

Recent studies have established a clear association between an everted labrum and the presence of hip dysplasia.[5,6] However, contrary to the characteristic hypertrophic labrum seen in the prototypical dysplastic hip, paradoxic labral hypoplasia is common in dysplasia with labral eversion.[3,5–9] This phenomenon is attributable to minimal or complete lack of shear force-induced reactive labral hyperplasia due to poor or absent femoral head apposition and shielding from stress. Given this association, it can be inferred that a number of patients with recurrent instability and/or pain following hip preservation surgery have an unaddressed everted labrum contributing to the continued symptomatic disease.[5,6]

An everted labrum is a frequently overlooked pathology, as surgeons must have prior understanding to specifically look for the characteristic findings preoperatively and then confirm diagnosis intraoperatively in order to intervene appropriately. Several characteristic preoperative imaging findings are highly associated with an everted labrum. On MRI, a gap between the labrum and femoral head, labral hypoplasia, and a blunted labral shape are correlated with labral eversion (**Fig. 1**A–D). Further,

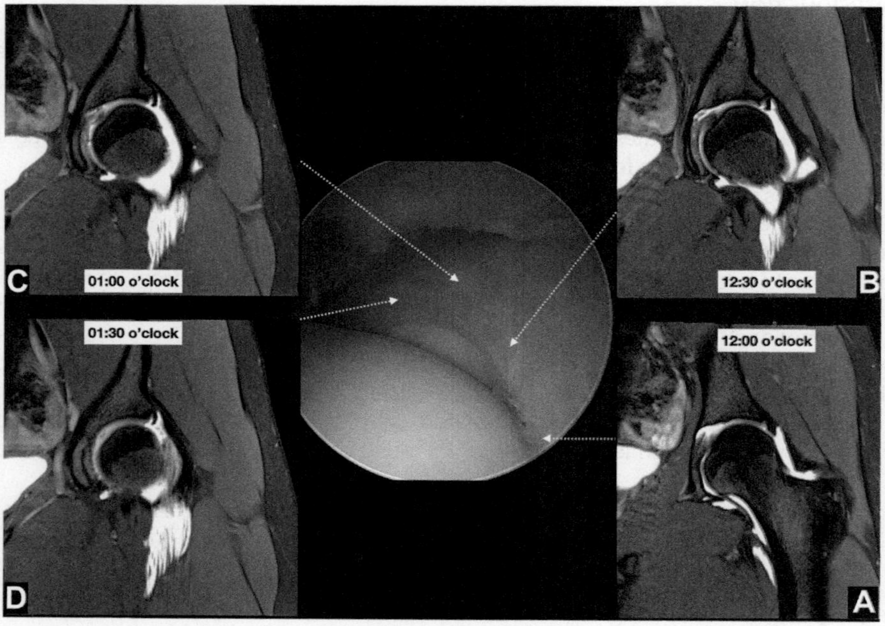

Fig. 1. (*A–D*) An arthroscopic image from a left hip with traction removed in the center image, with the hip in the neutral/extended position before any work was done, with corresponding clock-face position coronal T2 fat-saturated MR images. The native labrum lacks direct contact with the femoral head, demonstrating an everted acetabular labrum.

identification of an upsloping sourcil observed on weight-bearing plain radiographs, or advanced imaging, commonly recognized as a morphologic variant of acetabular dysplasia, is associated with an everted labrum (**Fig. 2**A–D).[5,6] However, with these preoperative imaging findings, sensitivity in diagnosis is yet to be established. As noted in the first article to characterize the native everted labrum by Vogel and colleagues,[6] everted labrum patients demonstrated significantly larger labrum-femoral head distance, with a significantly greater proportion of patients demonstrating a blunted or round labral shape. However, every everted labrum cannot be reliably diagnosed with preoperative imaging, thus intraoperative confirmation is always required.

Definitive diagnosis must be made intraoperatively during hip arthroscopy.[5,6] Upon initial intraoperative arthroscopic evaluation of the acetabulum and labrum on traction, suspicion should be raised for labral eversion if superomedial sloping acetabular cartilage beneath the labrum is encountered (see **Fig. 2**). Diagnosis is confirmed when gapping (ie, lack of observed labral-femoral head contact) between the femoral head and labrum is encountered with hip traction completely removed. If suspected, meticulous evaluation without hip distraction is warranted, as confirmatory findings are often subtle and/or localized to a specific area, most commonly located anterolaterally. Thus,

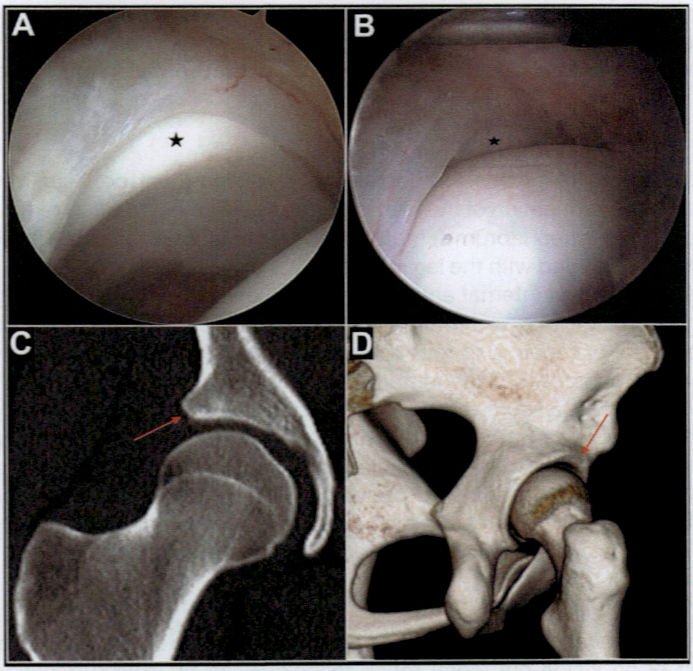

Fig. 2. Arthroscopic images of a right hip viewed through a midtrochanteric portal (*A* and *B*). (*A*) Arthroscopic image of a right hip with the hip on traction. The star indicates the articular cartilage lip that slopes from inferolateral to superomedial (seen on imaging as an upsloping sourcil) that is visible in the presence of labral eversion. (*B*) Arthroscopic image of the same right hip off of traction. Gapping between the labrum and femoral head visualized. The star indicates the same articular cartilage lip. (*C*) Coronal CT slice of the same hip with the *red arrow* demonstrating an up-slope[11]/lip that corresponds with the arthroscopic images (up-slope = exposed cartilage lip). This defines the area that serves as the labral bony footprint and that lacks weight-bearing contact with the femoral head. (*D*) 3D reconstruction of the same hip demonstrating the up-sloping area represented by the *red arrow*.

detailed evaluation utilizing multiple angles from both portals may be required for diagnosis.

It is instrumental to understand that an everted labrum can be an isolated, stand alone, diagnosis that results in symptomatic hip dysfunction without concomitant pathology such as dysplasia or femoracetabular impingement (FAI).[5,6] Thus, the presence of an everted labrum warrants surgical treatment to restore the acetabular suction seal. However, these patients frequently present with hip pain and concomitant pathologies that prompt surgeons to pursue surgical management. If an everted labrum is not recognized and treated during arthroscopic management of other pathologies, symptomatic disease will persist postoperatively due to the untreated dysfunctional suction seal. Similarly, when the labrum is iatrogenically everted or debrided rather than repaired, the suction seal can be unintentionally rendered functionally incompetent, leading to similar consequences as a native everted labrum. Insight into this theory can be evidenced by literature detailing a higher incidence of treatment failure in hips with hypoplastic labra undergoing arthroscopic labral repair.[10] Given the characteristic feature of labral hypoplasia in everted labra, it can intuitively be implied that at least a subset of these patients had an undiagnosed everted labrum contributing to postoperative treatment failure, as the "labral repair" lacked formal advancement and verification of appropriate labral-femoral head contact with the hip off traction. Therefore, education regarding proper identification of relevant pathology and appropriate operative indications and techniques would lead to improved postoperative patient outcomes.

EVERTED LABRUM REPAIR TECHNIQUE

During arthroscopy, diagnosis and location of eversion must be visualized prior to repair. Thorough examination of the joint is performed with hip traction removed. Diagnosis is confirmed when labrum-femoral head gapping is visualized with the hip off traction. This is observed with the leg in resting position (extension). It is also important to observe the effect of internal and external rotation of the hip as the magnitude of gapping may change due to femoral head asphericity. Once diagnosis confirmed, the principal goal of repair is to mobilize, or advance, the everted portion of labrum and bring it into contact with the femoral head to restore the suction seal. However, the method to achieve labrum-femoral head contact depends on the quantity of viable labral tissue available for mobilization and repair. If an adequate amount of viable labral tissue is present after careful capsule-labral separation is completed, an arthroscopic labral advancement with or without refixation should be performed. However, treatment with arthroscopic labral augmentation or construction may be unavoidable in the setting of deficient viable labrum to permit repair.

Labral Advancement and Repair

While numerous labral repair techniques are described in the literature,[8] our preference is utilization of an inside-out labral repair technique, as previously described.[11] This technique expediates optimal labral positioning through utilization of intra-articular suture anchor placement, which creates the required inferior pull on the labrum (**Fig. 3**A–D). This suture anchor placement produces an advantageous force vector to encourage approximation of the labrum to the femoral head. This is in contrast to traditional labral repair techniques, where the labrum experiences a superior pull from suture anchors, encouraging separation of the labrum from the head superiorly.

Following examination and identification of an everted labrum, mobilization of the labrum should be performed. This is better done off traction to relax the capsule and improve access to capsule-labral cleft. First, the surgeon separates the labrum

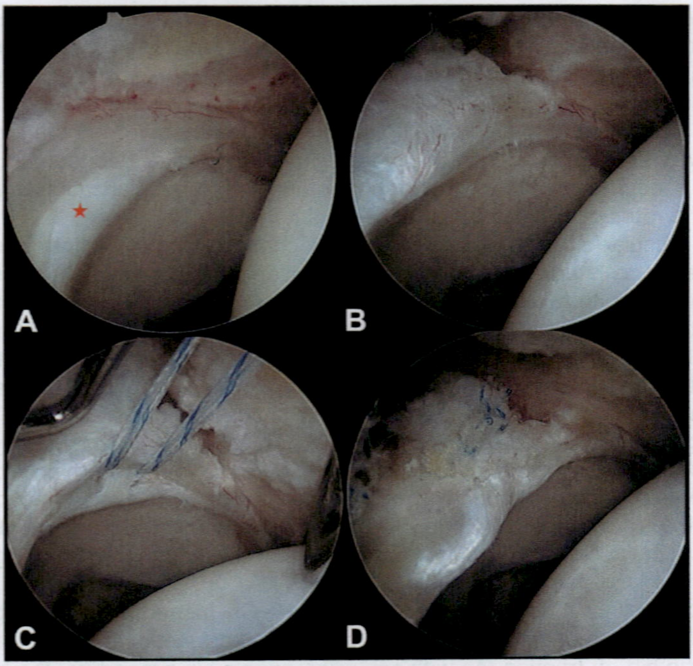

Fig. 3. Arthroscopic images of a right hip during an everted labrum advancement with an inside-out labral repair technique, viewed through a midtrochanteric portal. (*A*) Arthroscopic image of a right hip with the hip distracted. An articular cartilage lip beneath the labrum is demonstrated by the red star. (*B*) Arthroscopic image of the same hip after labral advancement. (*C*) An inside-out labral repair is performed so the vector of the suture anchor knots optimizes positioning of the labrum toward the femoral head. (*D*) Final view after labral advancement and repair, demonstrating that the articular cartilage lip is no longer visible.

and capsule in the area of eversion with electrocautery beginning at the apex of eversion (commonly at the 1 o'clock position), usually with a 30° arthroscope through an anterior portal and the cautery through the midtrochanteric portal. The portion of everted labrum must subsequently be fully released, employing caution to preserve labral tissue volume and viability. In hips presenting with significant distance between the labrum and femoral head, thin labral tissue, a large cartilage lip, or significant pincer pathology, an acetabuloplasty may be required to bring the labral foot-print closer to the femoral head and ensure contact prior to repair. In the presence of an articular cartilage lip, acetabuloplasty is typically carried out to the angle between the acetabular roof and the cartilage lip, in order for the labrum to be advanced from the upsloping sourcil portion toward its true footprint on the acetabular rim.[12] However, surgeons should be aware that this may have fully detached a portion of labrum creating a "flail" labrum, which must be addressed later in repair.

Once the labrum is mobilized with or without acetabuloplasty, surgeons should confirm that the advanced labrum contacts the femoral head with traction removed. Some cases may require advancement of only a small region, leaving a circumferentially intact chondro-labral junction with maintained overall labral stability. Retained labral integrity and stability obviates labral refixation, and, thus, a formal repair is generally not pursued in these cases.

Once the labrum can be freely mobilized with a probe at the chondro-labral junction, an inside-out labral repair can be performed. To begin repair, any reactive tissue and/or tearing is first debrided with a fine shaver (Double Bite, Stryker, small blade opening) or radiofrequency wand (S&N, Arthrocare 30°), and the acetabular rim edge at the site of anchor placement is rasped (ball tip, Arthrex) or gently burred in the presence of large uneven rim calcifications. The bleeding occurring after debridement provides an added benefit to healing through the facilitation of revascularization but can also increase the rates of capsule-labral adhesions.

On the articular side of the labrum at the chondro-labral junction, anchors are placed medial to lateral utilizing a firm angled drill guide with a distal curve, and c-arm verification, to avoid subchondral penetration. If located anteriorly around the 3 o'clock position, it is important to aim the drill guide posteriorly to avoid placement of the anchor beneath the iliopsoas, which may lead to postoperative irritation. After placement of the anchor, an arthroscopic suture passer is utilized for retrieval of both suture limbs through the labrum, which should be performed in a mattress manner, to the capsular side of the labrum. The labrum is then consequently secured via a standard arthroscopic knot tied from the apex of the eversion, which is thought to augment the advancement during repair. Sutures may be tied on or off traction. Suture tying with the hip distracted is beneficial because this enables for past-pointing; however, it is critical to first verify optimal repair position off traction by mimicking knot position with the knot-pusher.

After conclusion of labral refixation (**Fig. 4**A–C), inspection of the peripheral compartment ensures, with confirmation of a restored functional acetabular suction seal with the hip off traction. As with any arthroscopic hip procedure, the hip is then accessed for impingement necessitating femoral osteoplasty. Finally, the capsule is repaired, if possible, at the conclusion of the procedure.

Labral Augmentation or Reconstruction

When there is inadequate viable tissue available for repair after labral advancement, augmentation or reconstruction must be performed.[6] Surgeons should elect to proceed with labral reconstruction when remaining labral tissue is of low quality, prompting subsequent debridement and reconstruction with either allograft or autograft. Both allograft[13–16] and autograft[17–20] have proven efficacy, without demonstration of significant differences in patient outcomes between the 2 graft types.[21,22] While literature has demonstrated negligible differences between labral reconstruction and primary repair, primary repair should always be utilized first, if adequate healthy labrum tissue

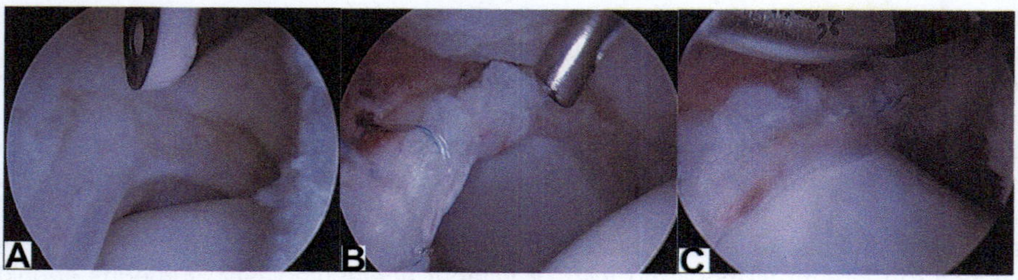

Fig. 4. Arthroscopic images of a right hip during inside-out arthroscopic labral repair viewed from a midtrochanteric portal. (*A*) Arthroscopic image of an everted labrum with the hip off traction, seen as gapping between the labrum and femoral head; (*B*) Arthroscopic image taken during labral advancement[10] showing the labrum covering the cartilage lip. (*C*) Arthroscopic image following everted labral repair, off traction, demonstrating a restoration of the fluid seal through restoration of labrum-femoral head contact.

presents for repair, as it is the current gold standard and results in lower rates of capsule-labral adhesions.[18,23]

For segmental reconstruction, the poor-quality labral tissue should be debrided, leaving behind healthy edges to permit a robust side-to-side anastomosis with the graft. Attention is then turned to the acetabular rim, where the surgeon should create a slightly upsloping bleeding rim surface, while ensuring that no weight-bearing bone is removed if stability is in question. This surface is optimal for graft healing and anatomic positioning. Then, utilizing an instrument with a known size, such as a probe, or designated arthroscopic ruler, the length of the defect is measured carefully in order to avoid a graft-defect size mismatch. With 6 to 8 mm spacing, suture anchors should be placed close to the cartilage edge to prevent graft eversion. An additional superior or anterior portal may be necessary for suture management. While the surgeon directs attention to additional work within the central or peripheral compartment, an assistant may prepare the graft. Our preferred allograft is either iliotibial band or tensor fascia lata, as it allows for simple adjustment of the graft diameter intraoperatively.[14] The graft should be sized around 110% of the measured defect, creating a few millimeters of graft-labrum overlap on both ends. The suture limbs from the most anterior and posterior anchors can be passed through the graft with a Keith needle outside of the joint and then the graft shuttled into the joint with a knot pusher employing a "kite" technique. Once the graft ends are secured on either side, the remaining suture anchors can then be passed around the graft one by one. After passing all sutures, knot tying should be performed. The anastomosis between the graft and native labrum typically occurs through suture anchor positioning behind the native labral tissue, negating the need for formal side by side anastomosis. It is critical to ensure graft security and position, as well as a functional suction seal with the hip off traction.

Augmentation is often selected, rather than complete native tissue resection and subsequent reconstruction, if there is insufficient tissue available for repair, but the remaining labral tissue still appears viable. Augmentation permits for the preservation of the circumferential native labral fibers and results in graft incorporation with the native labral tissue.[14,24] This preservation of native labral tissue enhances labral healing. This is favored over reconstruction when the labral tissue is amenable to augmentation. Labral augmentation is performed utilizing the same technique as the aforementioned labral reconstruction. The circumferential sutures are deployed to secure both graft and native labrum together.

DISCUSSION

The native everted labrum is a pathologic native variant warranting surgical management to restore the absent acetabular suction seal. It was shown that large cohorts of patients who fail surgical management of other concomitant hip pathology (such as labral repair, FAI, and so forth) have an unaddressed everted labrum leading to continued symptomatic disease. To evidence this, a recent analysis demonstrated significantly lower preoperative patient reported outcomes in patients with an everted labrum compared to a control group of preoperative patients.[5] These findings insinuate that persistent suction seal disruption due to an everted labrum potentiates hip pain from other pathologies. Of note, the aforementioned study described an isolated diagnosis of an everted labrum in 11.7% (n = 15) of the everted labrum cohort, suggesting that suction seal compromise alone is enough to cause symptomatic disease. Thus, an unrecognized everted labrum likely compromises arthroscopy success in many patients, stressing the importance of diligent analysis with the hip off traction during arthroscopy and expanding arthroscopic indications beyond FAI and dysplasia pathologies alone.

The benefit of surgical intervention with labral advancement or reconstruction/augmentation of the everted labrum is clear in practice. This clinical benefit was recently described in an article that analyzed the outcomes of surgical management for a cohort of 96 hips with an everted labrum.[5] The majority of the cohort underwent arthroscopic labral advancement (90.6%), while 10.4% were treated with labral reconstruction/augmentation. The study cohort demonstrated significant improvements in postoperative function, comparable to a control group despite lower preoperative values. Further, arthroscopic management for an everted labrum as the sole diagnosis yielded significant improvements in patient-reported outcome scores, indicating benefit of surgical management in the absence of other, more commonly diagnosed, hip pathology.

Further, we believe a key to successful management of hip instability and/or pain is addressing both soft tissue and bony contributors to symptomatic hip disease. The association of hip dysplasia and labral eversion, or hypoplastic nonfunctional labrum, is clear in the literature.[5,24] Although the pathogenesis of this association remains unclear, this is probably due to labral growth correspondent with an upsloping sourcil seen in dysplasia.[12] Surgical treatment of all amenable hip pathologies is our traditional approach to these patients, typically with a staged hip arthroscopy followed by periacetabular osteotomy (PAO) 1 to 2 weeks later.[25] Failure to address either the everted labrum arthroscopically or dysplasia via PAO would likely fail to improve long-term function. Several studies demonstrate poor efficacy in treating dysplasia with arthroscopic management alone, as persistent instability results in ongoing pain and damages the repaired soft tissues over time. The same referenced study on outcomes of surgical management of everted labra included 29 patients who underwent subsequent PAO for the management of concurrent hip dysplasia.[2] This everted labrum cohort reported significant improvement in postoperative function after their staged treatment of both soft tissue and bony pathologies. Further, a subanalysis comparing this cohort to patients with everted labrum and hip dysplasia who opted for arthroscopic management alone revealed significantly greater improvements in PROs in those managed with staged arthroscopy and PAO. This highlights the effectiveness of surgical management of everted labra in the setting of hip dysplasia and emphasizes the need to address all pathology contributing to symptomatic disease to optimize patient outcomes.

Surgeons must remain flexible regarding traditional management and techniques when confronted with an everted labrum. Conventional suture anchor placement generates a superior deviation of the labrum, which is undesirable in the setting of a compromised suction seal. This superiorly directed pull on the labrum worsens the labral pathoanatomy by pulling it further from anatomic position, preventing contact with the femoral head responsible for generation of the suction seal, even if labrum was advanced appropriately. Anchor placement is a small but critical variable to technical success and achieving functional improvement postoperatively.[26] Among other benefits the inside-out labral repair, it generates favorable force vectors to encourage apposition of the labrum to the femoral head, specifically advantageous when attempting to restore the suction seal. When anchors are placed away from the cartilage edge, the direction of pull can result in an iatrogenic everted labrum, even in cases without eversion preoperatively. Despite its technical difficulty, we believe the technique to be superior to conventional repair in the setting of suction seal compromise and believe surgeons should consider this in all cases involving a compromised acetabular suction seal.

Future Advancements

Further study is warranted regarding the native everted acetabular labrum. The origin of the everted labrum remains unclear. A greater understanding of its pathogenesis may aid early diagnosis and improvements in surgical treatment. Additionally, further studies addressing preoperative identification of an everted labrum would be beneficial, as without the practiced skill of recognizing the characteristic MRI findings, it cannot be reliably diagnosed until intraoperative inspection with the hip off traction. The association between multiple associated pathologies, such as hip dysplasia and the recently characterized Windshield Wiper Lesion, requires further inquiry to delineate the most effective treatment algorithms and techniques.[27] Finally, it is critical to continue expanding awareness of these challenging labral variants, as everted labra are frequently overlooked, precluding treatment that would significantly benefit patient function and satisfaction postoperatively.

SUMMARY

The everted labrum is a native labral variant that is diagnosed arthroscopically by gapping between the labrum and femoral head with the hip off traction. This is a pathologic condition characterized by hip pain and instability generated by disruption of the acetabular suction seal. When identified, restoration of the suction seal is the central goal of treatment. Arthroscopic treatment with labral advancement, augmentation, or reconstruction significantly improves patient-reported outcomes. It is necessary to correct both bony and soft tissue pathology leading to symptomatic disease to consistently achieve long-term postoperative improvements in patient function and satisfaction.

CLINICS CARE POINTS

- An everted labrum can be a stand-alone diagnosis causing symptomatic disease.
- Without prior knowledge to identify the characteristic findings, it is a commonly missed diagnosis.
- Definitively diagnosed arthroscopically, seen as gapping between the labrum and femoral head.
- Treatment consists of arthroscopic labral advancement, augmentation, or reconstruction with the goal of restoration of the suction seal.
- Inside-out labral repair technique is the preferred fixation method due to advantageous force vectors on the labrum from the suture anchors.
- Consider correction of any other concomitant bony and/or soft tissue abnormalities.

REFERENCES

1. Nepple JJ, Philippon MJ, Campbell KJ, et al. The hip fluid seal–Part II: the effect of an acetabular labral tear, repair, resection, and reconstruction on hip stability to distraction. Knee Surg Sports Traumatol Arthrosc 2014;22(4):730–6. PMID: 24509878.
2. Cadet ER, Chan AK, Vorys GC, et al. Investigation of the preservation of the fluid seal effect in the repaired, partially resected, and reconstructed acetabular labrum in a cadaveric hip model. Am J Sports Med 2012;40(10):2218–23. PMID: 22962293.
3. Petersen BD, Wolf B, Lambert JR, et al. Lateral acetabular labral length is inversely related to acetabular coverage as measured by lateral center edge angle of Wiberg. J Hip Preserv Surg 2016;3(3):190–6. PMID: 27583157.

4. Ross JR, Zaltz I, Nepple JJ, et al. Arthroscopic disease classification and interventions as an adjunct in the treatment of acetabular dysplasia. Am J Sports Med 2011;39(Suppl):72S–8S. PMID: 21709035.
5. Girardi NG, Lee JH, Genuario JW, et al. The everted acetabular labrum: outcomes of surgical management. Am J Sports Med 2024;52(6):1563–71. PMID: 38544383.
6. Vogel LA, Kraeutler MJ, Jesse MK, et al. The everted acetabular labrum: pathoanatomy, magnetic resonance imaging and arthroscopic findings of a native variant. Arthroscopy 2022;38(1):72–9. PMID: 33957213.
7. Garabekyan T, Ashwell Z, Chadayammuri V, et al. Lateral acetabular coverage predicts the size of the hip labrum. Am J Sports Med 2016;44(6):1582–9. PMID: 26989071.
8. Kraeutler MJ, Garabekyan T, Pascual-Garrido C, et al. Hip instability: a review of hip dysplasia and other contributing factors. Muscles Ligaments Tendons J 2016; 6(3):343–53. PMID: 28066739.
9. Kraeutler MJ, Safran MR, Scillia AJ, et al. A contemporary look at the evaluation and treatment of adult borderline and frank hip dysplasia. Am J Sports Med 2020; 48(9):2314–23. PMID: 31725329.
10. Kaplan DJ, Samim M, Burke CJ, et al. Decreased hip labral width measured via preoperative magnetic resonance imaging is associated with inferior outcomes for arthroscopic labral repair for femoroacetabular impingement. Arthroscopy 2021;37(1):98–107. PMID: 32828937.
11. Mei-Dan O, Pascual-Garrido C, Kark JA, et al. Inside out: a novel labral repair and advancement technique. Arthrosc Tech 2014;3(2):e241–4. PMID: 24904768.
12. Wong TY, Jesse MK, Jensen A, et al. Upsloping lateral sourcil: a radiographic finding of hip instability. J Hip Preserv Surg 2018;5(4):435–42. PMID: 30647935.
13. Carreira DS, Kruchten MC, Emmons BR, et al. Arthroscopic labral reconstruction using fascia lata allograft: shuttle technique and minimum two-year results. J Hip Preserv Surg 2018;5(3):247–58. PMID: 30393552.
14. McConkey MO, Moreira B, Mei-Dan O. Arthroscopic hip labral reconstruction and augmentation using knotless anchors. Arthrosc Tech 2015;4(6):e701–5. PMID: 26870649.
15. Rathi R, Mazek J. Arthroscopic acetabular labral reconstruction with Fascia Lata allograft: clinical outcomes at minimum one-year Follow-Up. Open Orthop J 2017; 11:554–61. PMID: 28839500.
16. White BJ, Stapleford AB, Hawkes TK, et al. Allograft use in arthroscopic labral reconstruction of the hip with front-to-back fixation technique: minimum 2-Year Follow-up. Arthroscopy 2016;32(1):26–32. PMID: 26422708.
17. Amar E, Sampson TG, Sharfman ZT, et al. Acetabular labral reconstruction using the indirect head of the rectus femoris tendon significantly improves patient reported outcomes. Knee Surg Sports Traumatol Arthrosc 2018;26(8):2512–8. PMID: 28717888.
18. Domb BG, El Bitar YF, Stake CE, et al. Arthroscopic labral reconstruction is superior to segmental resection for irreparable labral tears in the hip: a matched-pair controlled study with minimum 2-year follow-up. Am J Sports Med 2014;42(1): 122–30. PMID: 24186974.
19. Lebus GF, Briggs KK, Dornan GJ, et al. Acetabular labral reconstruction: development of a tool to predict outcomes. Am J Sports Med 2018;46(13):3119–26. PMID: 30285463.

20. Rathi R, Mazek J. Arthroscopic acetabular labral reconstruction with rectus femoris tendon autograft: our experiences and early results. J Orthop 2018;15(3): 783–6. PMID: 29997421.
21. Rahl MD, LaPorte C, Steinl GK, et al. Outcomes after arthroscopic hip labral reconstruction: a systematic review and meta-analysis. Am J Sports Med 2020; 48(7):1748–55. PMID: 31634004.
22. Lee S, Wuerz TH, Shewman E, et al. Labral reconstruction with iliotibial band autografts and semitendinosus allografts improves hip joint contact area and contact pressure: an in vitro analysis. Am J Sports Med 2015;43(1):98–104. PMID: 25361860.
23. Maldonado DR, Lall AC, Walker-Santiago R, et al. Hip labral reconstruction: consensus study on indications, graft type and technique among high-volume surgeons. J Hip Preserv Surg 2019;6(1):41–9. PMID: 31069094.
24. Philippon MJ, Bolia IK, Locks R, et al. Labral preservation: outcomes following labrum augmentation versus labrum reconstruction. Arthroscopy 2018;34(9): 2604–11. PMID: 30173800.
25. Mei-Dan O, Welton KL, Kraeutler MJ, et al. The CU PAO: a minimally invasive, 2-Incision, interlocking periacetabular osteotomy: technique and early results. J Bone Joint Surg Am 2019;101(16):1495–504. PMID: 31436658.
26. Degen RM, O'Sullivan E, Sink EL, et al. Psoas tunnel perforation-an unreported complication of hip arthroscopy. J Hip Preserv Surg 2015;2(3):272–9. PMID: 27011849.
27. Girardi NG, Kraeutler MJ, Jesse MK, et al. The windshield wiper sign is an instability-related osteochondral defect of the anterolateral femoral head. Arthroscopy 2025;41(4):927–36. PMID: 38697329.

Hip Labral Reconstruction

Lessons Learned from 1000 Cases

Ady H. Kahana-Rojkind, MD[a,b,c], Roger Quesada-Jimenez, MD[a], Benjamin G. Domb, MD[a,d,*]

KEYWORDS

- Hip arthroscopy • Labral reconstruction • Femoroacetabular impingement
- Allograft • Acetabuloplasty • Return to sport

KEY POINTS

- Labral repair remains the gold standard, but reconstruction is essential when the labrum is irreparable.
- The knotless pull-through technique streamlines graft passage, eliminates sizing, and allows reproducible fixation.
- Careful rim preparation, graft handling, and structured suture management are critical to optimizing outcomes.
- Reconstruction provides reliable improvements in patient-reported outcomes and return-to-sport rates, comparable to repair.
- Predictive factors such as age, body mass index, Tönnis grade, Lateral Center-Edge Angle (LCEA), and alpha angle can help anticipate the need for reconstruction.

Video content accompanies this article at http://www.sportsmed.theclinics.com.

INTRODUCTION

The acetabular labrum is a crucial component for the hip joint stability.[1] It maintains intra-articular pressurization, generating the negative pressure suction seal that contributes to joint stability.[2,3] Beyond this, the labrum increases acetabular volume by approximately 33%, deepening the socket, and enhances resistance to translational and rotational forces acting on the femoral head.[3–5]

Damage to the labrum, therefore, has significant biomechanical consequences, disrupting fluid pressurization, diminishing stability, and accelerating chondral degeneration.

[a] American Hip Institute Research Foundation, Chicago, IL, USA; [b] Department of Orthopaedic Surgery, ABC Medical Center, Mexico City, Mexico; [c] Ortomove, Mexico City, Mexico; [d] American Hip Institute, Chicago, IL, USA

* Corresponding author. American Hip Institute, 999 E Touhy Avenue, Suite 450, Des Plaines, IL 60018.

E-mail address: drdomb@americanhipinstitute.org

Clin Sports Med 45 (2026) 633–646
https://doi.org/10.1016/j.csm.2026.01.002 sportsmed.theclinics.com

Abbreviations	
AL	anterolateral
ASIS	anterior superior iliac spine
BMI	body mass index
DALA	distal anterolateral accessory
MA	midanterior
PL	posterolateral
PROs	patient-reported outcomes
THA	total hip arthroplasty

Hip arthroscopy has been shown to be an effective and reliable treatment of femoroacetabular impingement and labral tears, with well-documented long-term results. However, in cases of irreparable labral tears, labral reconstruction has been shown to be superior to other treatment options, such as segmental excision or debridement, to restore the biomechanics and function of the acetabular labrum, with favorable midterm and long-term outcomes in both primary and revision settings.[6–12] Although favorable outcomes have been widely reported, several series have also noted high rates of revision arthroscopy and eventual conversion to total hip arthroplasty (THA) in patients undergoing reconstruction, underscoring the importance of careful patient selection, meticulous surgical technique, and recognition of the steep learning curve associated with this procedure.[6,10,13–15]

Over the years, a range of reconstructive strategies—including labral augmentation, capsular advancement, and circumferential reconstruction—have been developed to address this challenge.[16,17] Among them, the knotless pull-through technique has proven reproducible and efficient, eliminating the need for intraoperative graft measurement while consistently restoring the suction seal.[12,18]

Drawing on experience from more than 1000 reconstructions, the senior author has identified key lessons spanning indications, technical pearls, and rehabilitation strategies. Together, these insights have improved reproducibility and clinical outcomes. The following sections detail the current technique for knotless pull-through labral reconstruction and summarize the lessons learned across a large consecutive series of patients.

INDICATIONS AND CONTRAINDICATIONS

Labral reconstruction is indicated when the native labrum is deemed irreparable and unable to contribute meaningfully to hip stability or suction seal restoration. Irreparability is defined intraoperatively by labral tissue measuring 2 mm or less in thickness, severe intrasubstance degeneration, extensive calcification, complex tearing with loss of the chondro-labral junction, or loss of viable tissue secondary to prior aggressive debridement or iatrogenic excision (**Table 1**).[19–21] Reconstruction is also frequently performed in revision settings when prior labral repair has failed, and nonviable tissue or excessive debridement precludes preservation of the labrum.[22] Because the determination of irreparability is made intraoperatively, labral reconstruction must be included in the preoperative consent process, and graft availability ensured, whenever a repair is planned. This ensures patients are appropriately counseled regarding the possibility of reconstruction and avoids the need for staged procedures.

Contraindications to labral reconstruction are primarily related to underlying hip pathology that limits the potential for meaningful recovery. Absolute contraindications include advanced osteoarthritis, that is, severe joint space narrowing (<2 mm) or Tönnis grade 2 or greater, as these patients are better served with arthroplasty.[16,23,24]

Table 1
Indications and contraindications for arthroscopic labral reconstruction

Indications	Contraindications
Labral tissue ≤2 mm in thickness	Advanced osteoarthritis (Tönnis grade ≥2)
Severe intrasubstance degeneration	Severe joint space narrowing (<2 mm)
Extensive labral calcification Segmental or circumferential defects	—
Complex tearing	—
Loss of viable tissue due to prior aggressive debridement or iatrogenic excision	—

Over the course of the senior author's experience, a critical lesson has been the importance of rigorous intraoperative assessment of labral tissue quality. Attempting to repair tissue that is calcified, insufficient, or structurally compromised often leads to suboptimal outcomes and subsequent revision surgery.[25,26] Establishing strict indications for reconstruction has, therefore, improved both technical consistency and patient outcomes.

GRAFT CHOICE

A wide range of grafts have been described for hip labral reconstruction, broadly categorized into autografts and allografts. The ideal graft should replicate the anatomy and function of the native labrum while minimizing morbidity, reducing operative time, and ensuring consistent handling. Patient factors, surgeon experience, availability, and cost all influence graft selection.[27]

Autografts, including iliotibial band, hamstring tendons, rectus femoris, and capsular tissue, have been widely reported with favorable results. A systematic review summarized outcomes from over 400 patients and demonstrated consistent improvements in functional scores, with low rates of revision and conversion to arthroplasty.[28] Advantages of autografts include biologic incorporation, independence from tissue bank availability, and lower cost. However, autograft harvest introduces donor-site morbidity, increases operative time, and may limit graft length, particularly in circumferential reconstructions.

Allografts—including tibialis anterior and posterior, iliotibial band, semitendinosus, and peroneus brevis—offer several advantages. Their morphology is often cylindrical, requiring minimal preparation, and they provide reproducible size and length, which is especially valuable in circumferential reconstructions. They also eliminate donor-site morbidity and decrease operative time. Comparative studies have generally shown no significant differences in outcomes between autografts and allografts (**Table 2**).[29,30] Though one series reported higher revision rates with allograft compared to autograft, while patient-reported outcomes, satisfaction, and conversion to THA rates were equivalent.[31]

From a technical perspective, the senior author's preference is for tibialis posterior allograft, which has proven the most efficient and dependable option. Its natural cylindrical morphology eliminates the need for tubularization, simplifying preparation and avoiding the additional suture material required for tubular grafts, which can act as a nidus for irritation or infection. Combined with the elimination of donor-site morbidity, reduction in operative time, and consistent graft handling, tibialis posterior

Table 2
Comparison of autograft and allograft options for hip labral reconstruction

Feature	Autograft	Allograft
Common sources	Iliotibial band, hamstrings, rectus femoris, ligamentum teres, hip capsule, and quadriceps	Tibialis posterior, tibialis anterior, iliotibial band, hamstrings, tensor fascia lata, and peroneus brevis
Advantages	• No risk of disease transmission • Readily available without tissue bank • Lower material cost	• No donor site morbidity • Eliminates harvest time • Consistent size/length—reliable handling
Disadvantages	• Donor site morbidity • Increased operative time • Limited graft length in some sources	• Higher cost • Requires tissue bank availability • Theoretic risk of disease transmission

allograft has become the preferred graft in our high-volume practice. Autografts remain a reliable alternative, particularly in cases where allograft tissue is not available, cost-prohibitive, or reconstruction is unexpectedly required intraoperatively.

SURGICAL TECHNIQUE

The patient is placed supine on a postless traction table under general anesthesia. Both feet are carefully padded, and the legs are positioned in neutral rotation. To optimize joint distraction and provide clear access to the central compartment, the operating table is tilted 10° to 15° in Trendelenburg.[32] Arthroscopic access is obtained through 4 standard portals: anterolateral (AL), midanterior (MA), distal anterolateral accessory (DALA), and posterolateral (PL; **Fig. 1**). The AL portal, created first under fluoroscopic guidance at the 12 o'clock position, serves as the primary viewing portal with a 70° arthroscope.[33] The MA and DALA portals provide working access for rim preparation and anchor placement. The PL portal is vital to the pull-through labral

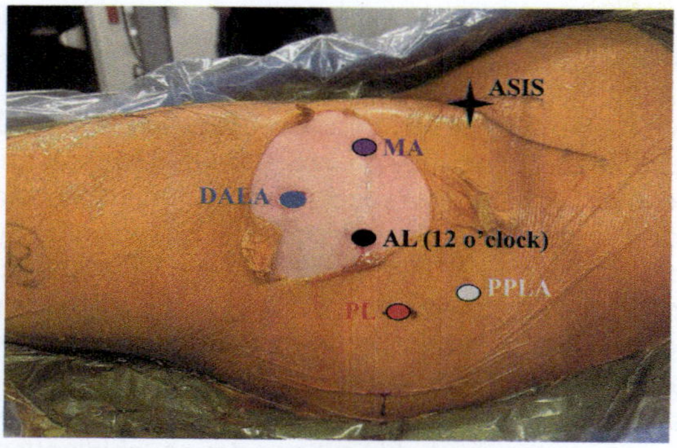

Fig. 1. Arthroscopic portals for labral reconstruction in a left hip. Landmarks include the anterior superior iliac spine (ASIS). Portals shown are anterolateral (AL, viewing portal at the 12 o'clock position), mid-anterior (MA), distal anterolateral accessory (DALA), and posterolateral (PL). A proximal posterolateral accessory (PPLA) portal may be used optionally to facilitate suture management. *Image Courtesy:* American Hip Institute.

reconstruction technique, as the posterior end of the graft is introduced through the DALA portal and retrieved through the PL portal. In addition, the PL portal is routinely used for anchor placement in the posterior acetabulum, providing the optimal trajectory for fixation in this region. In circumferential reconstructions requiring many anchors, an additional proximal posterolateral accessory portal may be established to improve suture management. Retrieving the posterior sutures through this accessory portal simplifies organization, keeps them from crossing through the arthroscopic field of view, and leaves the PL clear for drilling, which facilitates anchor placement in the more posterior acetabulum.

All nonviable labral tissue is meticulously debrided to stable margins using a radiofrequency probe and arthroscopic shaver. A burr is then employed to expose a bleeding bone surface and prepare the acetabular rim for graft fixation. Complete removal of degenerated tissue ensures an appropriate environment for graft incorporation, while decortication of the rim establishes a biologically favorable graft bed. Beyond simple debridement, beveling the rim to approximately 60° has proven to be an important refinement (**Fig. 2**).[34] This maneuver increases the surface area for graft contact and allows the reconstructed labrum to rest against the femoral head in an anatomic orientation, thereby optimizing the suction seal.[35] While contouring the rim, the burr is also used to deepen the psoas notch to adequately seat the first anchor in strong bone. Another important lesson has been the sequencing of steps. Any necessary femoroplasty is performed immediately after acetabular rim preparation and before graft passage. Leaving graft introduction and fixation as the final stage of the procedure eliminates the need to manage the graft while other work is ongoing and minimizes the time the graft remains submerged in solution, thereby reducing the risk of graft swelling.

Graft preparation is performed on the back table while rim work is being completed. A tibialis posterior allograft is preferred owing to its natural cylindrical shape, which eliminates the need for tubularization and makes preparation efficient and reproducible. The graft is sized to 6 to 7 mm in diameter, closely matching the native labrum. One end of the graft is reinforced with multiple Krackow stitches using 2.0 FiberLoop sutures, providing secure fixation and facilitating passage, while the opposite end is secured with a ripstop stitch to resist suture cut-through during fixation (**Fig. 3**). A

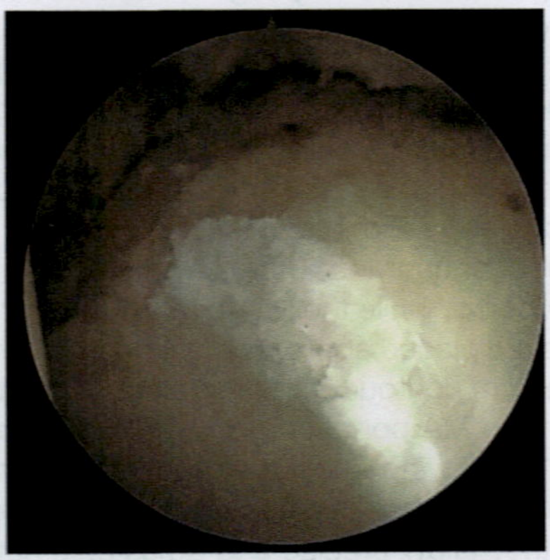

Fig. 2. Intraoperative arthroscopic image obtained from the anterolateral (AL) portal using a 70° arthroscope, demonstrating acetabular rim preparation prior to labral reconstruction. The rim has been contoured to a 60° bevel to optimize graft contact, facilitate anchor placement, and restore the suction seal. *Image Courtesy:* American Hip Institute.

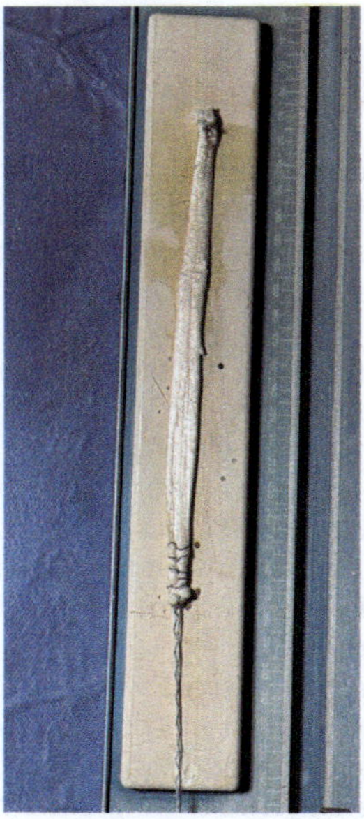

Fig. 3. Intraoperative photograph of posterior tibialis allograft preparation. The posterior end is reinforced with a Krackow stitch (*solid arrow*), while the anterior end is secured with a ripstop stitch (*dotted arrow*). *Image Courtesy:* American Hip Institute.

distinct advantage of the pull-through technique is that the graft does not need to be measured intraoperatively. Because it is prepared longer than the anticipated defect, the excess length is simply amputated at the conclusion of fixation, ensuring sufficiency without the need for sizing. For this reason, the distinction between segmental and circumferential reconstruction becomes less relevant, as the same technique reliably addresses both scenarios without the need for intraoperative length calculations. Once preparation is complete, the graft should not be left submerged in solution; instead, it is wrapped in gauze that is only slightly moistened, which maintains hydration while minimizing swelling prior to passage.

Following graft preparation, knotless all-suture anchors are placed sequentially from anterior to posterior along the acetabular rim to span the length of the reconstruction (**Fig. 4**A, B). The first 2 anchors are typically placed via the MA portal, which provides an optimal angle for fixation in the anterior acetabulum. To further ensure fixation strength at this critical point, the second anchor is placed very close to the first serving as a fail-safe in the event of anchor loosening. The remaining anchors are most often placed through the DALA portal, while the PL portal is used for anchors at the posterior extent of the rim. Anchors are placed approximately 6 mm apart, which provides secure fixation and ensures a uniform contour of the reconstructed labrum. Each set of suture limbs is retrieved through the MA portal and is organized clamped to the drape in the order they were placed, simplifying subsequent identification, fixation, and reducing the risk of confusion (**Fig. 5**). The use of all-suture knotless anchors has proven particularly advantageous, as they allow precise and adjustable suture tensioning, create a low-profile repair that minimizes articular cartilage irritation, reduce operative time through simplified fixation, and preserve bone stock owing to their smaller drill sites.

Once anchors are secured, the graft is introduced. The Krakow stitch sutures on the posterior end are inserted through the DALA portal and retrieved through the PL portal.

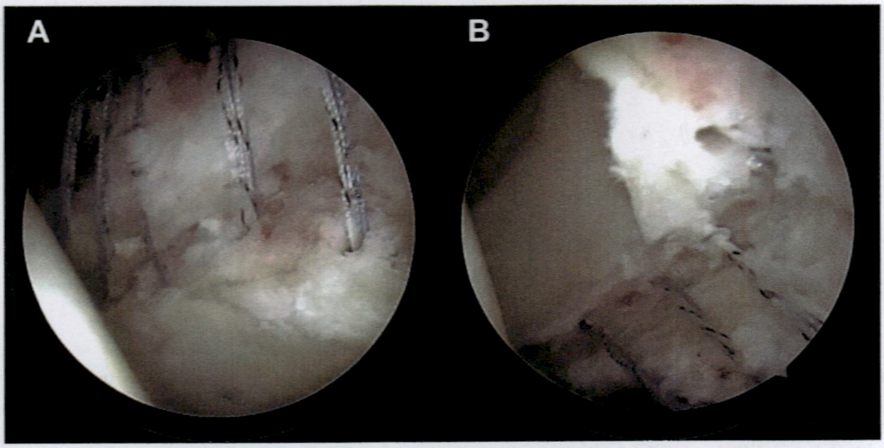

Fig. 4. Intraoperative arthroscopic images obtained from the anterolateral (AL) portal using a 70° arthroscope, demonstrating anchor placement during a circumferential labral reconstruction. (*A*) Anterior anchor placement. (*B*) Posterior anchor placement. *Image Courtesy:* American Hip Institute.

The most anterior anchor's repair suture is retrieved through the DALA portal and is passed through the graft adjacent to the ripstop stitch with a Keith needle. While holding the repair stich, the graft is pulled into the joint and out the PL portal, completing the pull-through maneuver (**Fig. 6**A, B). This step delivers the graft smoothly across the joint and into position along the prepared rim.

Fixation begins anteriorly, with a knot pusher through the DALA portal, the graft is advanced until it lies flush with the acetabular rim. The looped end of the shuttle suture is then retrieved from the same portal and connected to the repair suture. By pulling the opposite limb of the shuttle suture, the construct is tensioned, securely docking the graft at the first anchor site. The remaining anchors are then engaged sequentially from anterior to posterior, with each repair suture passed around the graft and secured using the knotless shuttle mechanism until the graft is fully seated along the rim

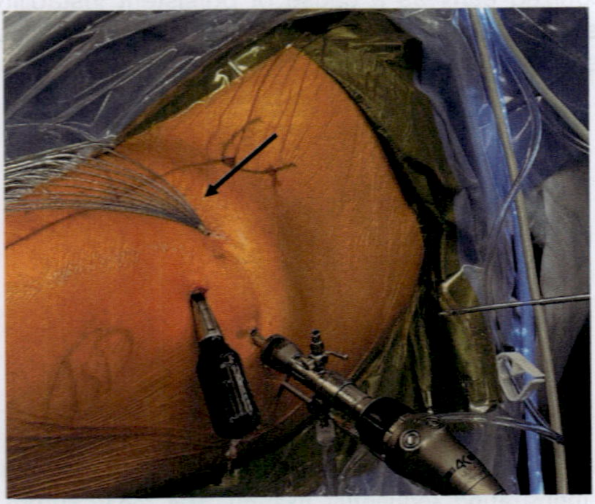

Fig. 5. Intraoperative image showing sutures retrieved through the midanterior (MA) portal (*black arrow*) and sequentially clamped to the drape to maintain organization and facilitate subsequent fixation. *Image Courtesy:* American Hip Institute.

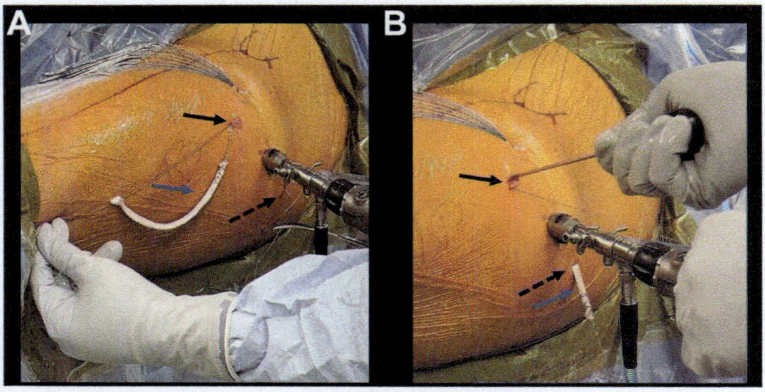

Fig. 6. Intraoperative images demonstrating the pull-through technique. (*A*) Initiation of graft passage, with the graft (*blue arrow*) being pulled into the distal anterolateral accessory (DALA) portal by tensioning the Krackow stitch that had been retrieved through the posterolateral (PL) portal (*dotted black arrow*). (*B*) Completion of passage, with the posterior end retrieved through the PL portal while the anterior end is seated into the first anchor via the mid-anterior (MA) portal (*solid black arrow*) using a knot pusher as the knotless mechanism is engaged. *Image Courtesy:* American Hip Institute.

(**Fig. 7**). A key refinement has been to apply traction on the graft through the PL portal before fully engaging the knotless mechanism at each anchor. This maneuver removes slack from the construct, ensures even seating of the graft, and prevents contour irregularities or bunching along the acetabular rim. Excess graft is amputated with a radiofrequency device to achieve a precise fit within the defect.

After fixation is completed, traction is released and dynamic arthroscopic evaluation is performed to confirm restoration of the suction seal and femoral head containment (**Fig. 8**). The reconstructed labrum should coapt smoothly against the femoral head throughout motion without excessive bulk (Video 1).

At the conclusion of the procedure, the capsule is routinely repaired. Simple closure is performed in most cases, with plication added when indicated, particularly in patients with capsular laxity or borderline dysplasia. Failure to adequately address the capsule was recognized early as a cause of persistent instability, even when the reconstruction itself was technically successful. Standardized closure has therefore become an integral part of the technique.

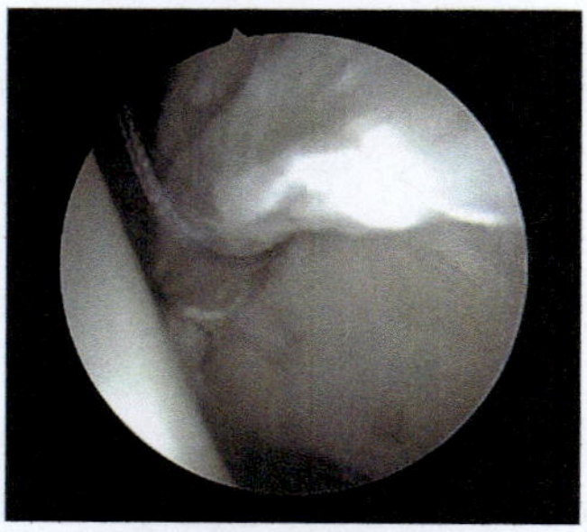

Fig. 7. Intraoperative arthroscopic image obtained from the anterolateral (AL) portal using a 70° arthroscope, demonstrating sequential fixation. The repair suture from the knotless anchor (*solid black arrow*) is passed around the graft (*dotted black arrow*), and tensioning the construct secures the graft to the acetabular rim. *Image Courtesy:* American Hip Institute.

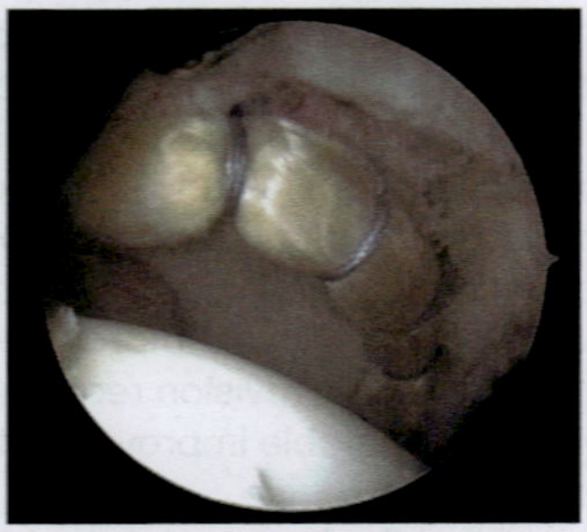

Fig. 8. Intraoperative arthroscopic image obtained from the anterolateral (AL) portal using a 70° arthroscope, showing the final construct after circumferential labral reconstruction. The graft is securely fixated to the acetabular rim, restoring the anatomic contour and suction seal. *Image Courtesy:* American Hip Institute.

Postoperatively, patients are placed in a hip brace to limit excessive motion. Weight-bearing is restricted to 20 pounds with crutches for 6 weeks. Physical therapy begins within 48 hours, emphasizing passive range of motion and stationary bicycling. At 6 weeks, therapy progresses to active strengthening, range-of-motion work, and stability training. Return to sport is guided by a structured protocol, including motion analysis at 6 months.

DISCUSSION/OUTCOMES

Arthroscopic labral reconstruction has become a reliable option in hip preservation surgery, consistently improving pain and function in patients with irreparable labral pathology. Systematic reviews confirm that reconstruction leads to significant improvement in patient-reported outcomes (PROs) and durable midterm to long-term survivorship.[36] Domb and colleagues,[37] in a nested matched-pair analysis with minimum 5 year follow-up, further demonstrated that reconstruction yields comparable improvements and survivorship to labral repair, establishing it as a clinically effective alternative when preservation is not possible.

Return to sport is particularly relevant for the young and athletic population. Jimenez and colleagues[38] showed that athletes undergoing primary reconstruction achieved high rates of return to sport at a median of 6 months, with results equivalent to a matched repair cohort. These findings reinforce that reconstruction, when repair is not feasible, does not compromise an athlete's ability to resume sport-specific training and competition.

Comparative studies highlight a treatment hierarchy. Maldonado and colleagues[39] found in a large systematic review that both repair and reconstruction produced substantial and clinically meaningful improvements, though reconstruction patients converted to THA at slightly higher rates. Complementing this, cadaveric biomechanical work showed that reconstruction does not surpass repair or the intact native labrum in restoring the suction seal, but consistently outperforms excision in maintaining distractive stability and fluid dynamics.[1] Collectively, these studies emphasize that repair should be prioritized when possible, but reconstruction is superior to debridement or excision and restores meaningful biomechanics when the labrum cannot be salvaged.

Patient selection is critical. Maldonado and colleagues[40] developed a predictive model from over 1300 hips, identifying older age, higher body mass index (BMI), Tönnis grade 1 or higher, larger LCEA, and increased alpha angle as predictors of requiring reconstruction. These findings reinforce the need for careful preoperative evaluation and for ensuring graft availability whenever repair is planned. Younger patients may also benefit: in a series of adolescents and young adults, significant improvements in PROs and high satisfaction were observed at 2 year follow-up, confirming the role of reconstruction even in early joint-preservation scenarios.[41]

In revision surgery, reconstruction is particularly valuable when tissue is deficient. Perets and colleagues[24] compared revision reconstruction with revision repair and found that both groups achieved significant improvement in PROs, with similar complication and reoperation rates. While revision repair achieved slightly higher final scores, reconstruction provided comparable improvement and remained an effective solution in the revision setting.

Taken together, the evidence and the lessons learned from over 1000 reconstructions highlight a consistent principle: In case of an irreparable labrum, labral reconstruction provides reproducible improvements in PROs, high return-to-sport rates, and survivorship.

SUMMARY

Labral reconstruction has become an integral option for managing irreparable labral tears, reliably improving pain, function, and return-to-sport rates when repair is not feasible. Although labral repair remains the gold standard when viable tissue is present, reconstruction provides durable survivorship and clinical outcomes superior to debridement or excision. Careful patient selection, meticulous rim preparation, reproducible graft handling, and structured rehabilitation are critical to optimizing results.

CLINICS CARE POINTS

- Repair when feasible: Preferred treatment when viable tissue is present; reconstruction indicated when irreparable.
- Reconstruction over excision: Superior outcomes compared with labral excision or debridement.
- Improved patient-reported outcomes: PROs reliably improve, with high satisfaction and survivorship comparable to repair.
- Return to sport restored: Athletes return at similar rates and timelines to repair.
- Predictive factors: Older age, higher BMI, Tönnis grade 1 or higher, larger LCEA, and higher alpha angle increase the likelihood of reconstruction.
- Allograft tissue, particularly tibialis posterior, is preferred to avoid donor site morbidity, reduce operative time.
- *Technical pearls*:
- Always ensure graft availability, even if the preoperative plan is labral repair, since irreparability is determined intraoperatively.
- Bevel rim to approximately 60° to optimize graft contact, suction seal, and anchor placement.
- Use knotless all-suture anchors for precise tensioning, low profile, and bone preservation.
- *Double-anchor anterior strategy*: Placing the first 2 anchors very close together (~3 mm apart) in the anterior acetabulum serves as a fail-safe against early anchor loosening.
- *Psoas notch preparation*: Deepen the notch to seat the first anchor securely in strong bone and avoid skiving.

- Retrieve and organize sutures sequentially through the MA portal to streamline organization.
- Apply gentle traction on the graft through the PL portal before engaging anchors to remove slack.
- *Pitfalls to avoid*:
- Excessive rim burring compromising femoral head coverage.
- Poor suture management leading to disorganization and technical difficulty.

DISCLOSURE

Dr A.H. Kahana-Rojkind reports receiving travel reimbursement from Arthrex, Stryker, and Zimmer Biomet. Dr R. Quesada-Jimenez reports receiving travel reimbursement from Arthrex, Stryker, and Zimmer Biomet. Dr B.G. Domb reports a relationship with Arthrex Inc that includes consulting or advisory, funding grants, nonfinancial support, speaking and lecture fees, royalties, and travel reimbursement; reports a relationship with DJO Global that includes royalties and nonfinancial support; reports a relationship with Medacta that includes royalties, consulting or advisory, and nonfinancial support; reports a relationship with Stryker that includes consulting or advisory, funding grants, nonfinancial support, and travel reimbursement; reports a relationship with Smith & Nephew that includes funding grants; reports a relationship with Orthomerica that includes royalties; reports a relationship with Medwest Associates Inc that includes nonfinancial support; reports a relationship with Ossur that includes funding grants; reports a relationship with Zimmer Biomet that includes nonfinancial support; reports a relationship with DePuy Synthes that includes nonfinancial support; reports a relationship with Medtronic that includes nonfinancial support; reports a relationship with SI-Bone, Inc. that includes consulting or advisory and nonfinancial support; reports a relationship with Trice Medical that includes nonfinancial support; reports a relationship with Xiros Inc. that includes nonfinancial support; reports a relationship with Intellijoint Surgical Inc. that includes nonfinancial support; reports a relationship with Electronic Waveform Lab, Inc. that includes nonfinancial support; has patent #8920497 with royalties paid from Arthrex; has patent #2612625 with royalties paid from Orthomerica and DJO Global; has patent #RE47811 with royalties paid from Arthrex; has patent #0338177 with royalties paid from Orthomerica. Dr B.G. Domb is a board member of American Hip Institute Research Foundation, AANA Learning Center Committee, the Journal of Hip Preservation Surgery, the Journal of Arthroscopy, AOSSM Research Committee, ISHA Executive Board; is Director of Hip Preservation at St. Alexius Medical Center; has had ownership interests in the American Hip Institute and affiliates, North Shore Surgical Suites, and Munster Specialty Surgery Center.

SUPPLEMENTARY DATA

Supplementary data related to this article can be found online at https://doi.org/10.1016/j.csm.2026.01.002.

REFERENCES

1. Maldonado DR, Owens JS, George T, et al. Acetabular labral reconstruction does not demonstrate superior biomechanical properties compared to labral repair or

intact native labrum but is superior to labral excision: a systematic review of cadaveric studies. Arthroscopy 2024;40(2):614–29.
2. Nogami R, Kaku N, Shimada T, et al. Three-dimensional architecture of the acetabular labrum in the human hip joint. Med Mol Morphol 2020;53(1):21–7.
3. Seldes RM, Tan V, Hunt J, et al. Anatomy, histologic features, and vascularity of the adult acetabular labrum. Clin Orthop 2001;382:232–40.
4. Hoffer AJ, Beel W, Ng KCG, et al. The contribution of soft tissue and bony stabilizers to the hip suction seal: a systematic review of biomechanical studies. Am J Sports Med 2024;52(10):2657–66.
5. Storaci HW, Utsunomiya H, Kemler BR, et al. The hip suction seal, part I: the role of acetabular labral height on hip distractive stability. Am J Sports Med 2020;48(11):2726–32.
6. Chandrasekaran S, Darwish N, Mu BH, et al. Arthroscopic reconstruction of the irreparable acetabular labrum: a match-controlled study. Arthroscopy 2019; 35(2):480–8.
7. Domb BG, El Bitar YF, Stake CE, et al. Arthroscopic labral reconstruction is superior to segmental resection for irreparable labral tears in the hip: a matched-pair controlled study with minimum 2-year follow-up. Am J Sports Med 2014;42(1): 122–30.
8. Domb BG, Hartigan DE, Perets I. Decision making for labral treatment in the hip: repair versus débridement versus reconstruction. J Am Acad Orthop Surg 2017; 25(3):e53–62.
9. Forster-Horvath C, Von Rotz N, Giordano BD, et al. Acetabular labral debridement/segmental resection versus reconstruction in the comprehensive treatment of symptomatic femoroacetabular impingement: a systematic review. Arthroscopy 2016;32(11):2401–15.
10. Maldonado DR, Kyin C, Shapira J, et al. Circumferential and segmental labral reconstruction: a systematic review. Orthopedics 2021;44(6):361–6.
11. Maldonado DR, Ouyang V, Lee MS, et al. After revision hip arthroscopy, patients having either circumferential or segmental labral reconstructions for the management of irreparable labra show clinical improvement based on proper indications. Arthroscopy 2022;38(8):2459–69.
12. Sabetian PW, Owens JS, Maldonado DR, et al. Circumferential and segmental arthroscopic labral reconstruction of the hip utilizing the knotless pull-through technique with all-suture anchors. Arthrosc Tech 2021;10(10):e2245–51.
13. Domb BG, Kyin C, Go CC, et al. Arthroscopic circumferential acetabular labral reconstruction for irreparable labra in the revision setting: patient-reported outcome scores and rate of achieving the minimal clinically important difference at a minimum 2-year follow-up. Am J Sports Med 2021;49(7):1750–8.
14. Domb BG, Prabhavalkar ON, Maldonado DR, et al. Long-term outcomes of arthroscopic labral treatment of femoroacetabular impingement in adolescents: a nested propensity-matched analysis. J Bone Jt Surg 2024;106(12):1062–8.
15. Litrenta JM, Mu BH, Chen AW, et al. Arthroscopic labral treatment in adolescents: clinical outcomes with minimum 5-year follow-up. Am J Sports Med 2019;47(4): 870–5.
16. Rosenthal RM, Featherall J, Parkes CW, et al. Acetabular labral reconstruction: review of techniques and outcomes. Curr Rev Musculoskelet Med 2023;16(10): 470–9.
17. Soares RW, Ruzbarsky JJ, Arner JW, et al. Midterm outcomes after hip labral augmentation in revision hip arthroscopy. Am J Sports Med 2022;50(5): 1299–305.

18. Perets I, Hartigan DE, Chaharbakhshi EO, et al. Circumferential labral reconstruction using the knotless pull-through technique—surgical technique. Arthrosc Tech 2017;6(3):e695–8.
19. Al Mana L, Coughlin RP, Desai V, et al. The hip labrum reconstruction: indications and outcomes—an updated systematic review. Curr Rev Musculoskelet Med 2019;12(2):156–65.
20. Maldonado DR, Lall AC, Walker-Santiago R, et al. Hip labral reconstruction: consensus study on indications, graft type and technique among high-volume surgeons. J Hip Preserv Surg 2019;6(1):41–9.
21. Jimenez AE, Lee MS, Owens JS, et al. Revision hip arthroscopy with labral reconstruction for irreparable labral tears in athletes: minimum 2-year outcomes with a benchmark control group. Am J Sports Med 2022;50(6):1571–81.
22. Shapira J, Kyin C, Go C, et al. Indications and outcomes of secondary hip procedures after failed hip arthroscopy: a systematic review. Arthroscopy 2020; 36(7):1992–2007.
23. Lameire DL, Pathak A, Hu SY, et al. The impact of hip arthroscopy on the progression of hip osteoarthritis in patients with femoroacetabular impingement syndrome: a systematic review and meta-analysis. Orthop J Sports Med 2025; 13(4):23259671251326116. https://doi.org/10.1177/23259671251326116.
24. Perets I, Rybalko D, Mu BH, et al. In revision hip arthroscopy, labral reconstruction can address a deficient labrum, but labral repair retains its role for the reparable labrum: a matched control study. Am J Sports Med 2018;46(14):3437–45.
25. Kahana-Rojkind AH, Rana K, Kingham YE, et al. Primary hip labral reconstruction shows superior outcomes compared with revision reconstruction after primary repair at minimum 2-year follow-up. Arthroscopy 2025;41(11):4583–93.e1.
26. Yuro MR, Kurapatti M, Carreira DS, et al. Secondary hip labral reconstruction yields inferior minimum 2-year functional outcomes to primary reconstruction despite comparable intraoperative labral characteristics. Arthroscopy 2024; 40(7):2009–17.
27. DeFroda SF, Hanish S, Muhammad M, et al. Graft options for hip labral reconstruction. JBJS Rev 2022;10(12):e22.00124. https://doi.org/10.2106/JBJS.RVW.22.00124.
28. Bessa FS, Williams BT, Polce EM, et al. Indications and outcomes for arthroscopic hip labral reconstruction with autografts: a systematic review. Front Surg 2020; 7:61.
29. Maldonado DR, Lall AC, Laseter JR, et al. Primary hip arthroscopic surgery with labral reconstruction: is there a difference between an autograft and allograft? Orthop J Sports Med 2019;7(3):2325967119833715. https://doi.org/10.1177/2325967119833715.
30. Rahl MD, LaPorte C, Steinl GK, et al. Outcomes after arthroscopic hip labral reconstruction: a systematic review and meta-analysis. Am J Sports Med 2020; 48(7):1748–55.
31. Cooper JD, Dekker TJ, Ruzbarsky JJ, et al. Autograft versus allograft: the evidence in hip labral reconstruction and augmentation. Am J Sports Med 2021;49-(13):3575–81.
32. Lall AC, Saadat AA, Battaglia MR, et al. Perineal pressure during hip arthroscopy is reduced by use of trendelenburg: a prospective study with randomized order of positioning. Clin Orthop 2019;477(8):1851–7.
33. Maldonado DR, Chen JW, Walker-Santiago R, et al. Forget the greater trochanter! hip joint access with the 12 o'clock portal in hip arthroscopy. Arthrosc Tech 2019; 8(6):e575–84.

34. Kahana-Rojkind AH, Keane JC, Kingham YE, et al. The beveled rim technique for labral reconstruction. Arthrosc Tech 2025;14(1):103156. https://doi.org/10.1016/j.eats.2024.103156.
35. Lall AC, Smith BL, Kahana-Rojkind AH, et al. Circumferential labral reconstruction with knotless all-suture anchors restores hip distractive stability: a cadaveric biomechanical analysis. Am J Sports Med 2024;52(14):3611–7.
36. Curley AJ, Padmanabhan S, Prabhavalkar ON, et al. Durable outcomes after hip labral reconstruction at minimum 5-year follow-up: a systematic review. Arthroscopy 2023;39(7):1702–13.
37. Domb BG, Battaglia MR, Perets I, et al. Minimum 5-year outcomes of arthroscopic hip labral reconstruction with nested matched-pair benchmarking against a labral repair control group. Am J Sports Med 2019;47(9):2045–55.
38. Jimenez AE, Monahan PF, Owens JS, et al. Return to sports and minimum 2-year outcomes of primary arthroscopic hip labral reconstruction for irreparable tears in high-level athletes with a propensity-matched benchmarking against a labral repair control group. Am J Sports Med 2021;49(12):3261–9.
39. Maldonado DR, Kyin C, Chen SL, et al. In search of labral restoration function with hip arthroscopy: outcomes of hip labral reconstruction versus labral repair: a systematic review. HIP Int 2021;31(6):704–13.
40. Maldonado DR, Chen JW, Walker-Santiago R, et al. Radiographic and demographic factors can predict the need for primary labral reconstruction in hip arthroscopic surgery: a predictive model using 1398 hips. Am J Sports Med 2020;48(1):173–80.
41. Maldonado DR, Glein RM, Saks BR, et al. Minimum 2-year outcomes following arthroscopic hip labral reconstruction in adolescents and young adults. J Pediatr Orthop 2022;42(2):83–9.

Advanced Femoral Osteochondroplasty: Achieving 2-Tier Sphericity and Symmetry

Jason G. Ina, MD[a,b,*], John M. Kopriva, MD[a],
Michael J. Salata, MD[a]

KEYWORDS

• Hip arthroscopy • Cam morphology • Femoroacetabular impingement

KEY POINTS

- Femoroacetabular impingement with cam morphology can be due to numerous etiologies and each presents with its own unique characteristics that influence impingement patterns and patient symptoms.
- Cam morphology is a 3-dimensional pathology that can be assessed with multiple 2-dimensional radiographs or cross-sectional imaging to provide a comprehensive assessment of spatial pathoanatomy.
- Alpha angle and femoral head-neck offset ratio remain poor predictors of postoperative outcomes. The reflection index incorporates both femoral head sphericity and offset and may better predict outcomes.

INTRODUCTION

Femoroacetabular impingement (FAI) is one of the most common causes of hip pain, with increasing incidence of FAI exhibited over the past 2 decades.[1] FAI can be secondary to cam morphology of the proximal femur, pincer morphology of the acetabulum, or a combination of the two. The irregular cam morphology of the proximal femur leads to premature impingement between the proximal femur and acetabulum through hip range of motion. Repetitive impingement over time results in progressive chondrolabral injury, and in the long term, potential subsequent osteoarthritis.[2]

Hip arthroscopy is often performed in the setting of failed nonoperative management for FAI given its low complication rate, favorable outcomes, and potential to delay the natural history of osteoarthritis.[3–5] Similar to the increasing incidence of

[a] Department of Orthopaedic Surgery, University Hospitals Drusinsky Sports Medicine Institute, Cleveland, OH, USA; [b] Rainbow Babies and Children, University Hospitals, Cleveland, OH, USA
* Corresponding author.
E-mail address: ina.jason@outlook.com

Clin Sports Med 45 (2026) 647–661
https://doi.org/10.1016/j.csm.2026.03.007 sportsmed.theclinics.com
0278-5919/26/

Abbreviations	
3D	3-dimensional
AL	anterolateral
FAI	femoroacetabular impingement
LCPD	Legg–Calve–Perthes disease
MAP	midanterior portal
mHHS	modified Harris Hip Score
RI	reflection index
SCFE	slipped capital femoral epiphysis
US	ultrasonography

FAI, hip arthroscopy has seen an increase in use over the past decade, with substantial continued projected growth.[6] Despite its increasing popularity, the failure rate of hip arthroscopy remains relatively high, with reported failure rates as high as 15.1% and revision rates ranging from 3.8% to 4.5%.[7,8] A notable risk factor for failure of hip arthroscopy is inadequate resection, including both over-resection and under-resection.[9–11] The goal of the proximal femoral osteoplasty in hip arthroscopy is restoration of femoral head sphericity and femoral head–neck offset. While radiographic parameters such as alpha angle and head–neck offset ratio have been successful at identifying and diagnosing cam lesion, their ability to predict postoperative outcomes is limited.[10,12–16] The lack of correlation between established radiographic measurements and postoperative outcomes makes surgical planning for an adequate cam resection challenging.

The purpose of this article is to highlight the etiology and imaging assessment of cam-type FAI as well as review outcomes as they relate to established cam resection parameters. With a thorough understanding of cam morphology and how various parameters influence outcomes, one can better plan their intraoperative cam resection to best restore native femoral head sphericity and femoral head–neck offset.

ETIOLOGY OF CAM MORPHOLOGY

Cam morphology was initially described as a *pistol grip deformity* of the proximal femur with decreased sphericity and femoral head–neck offset when compared to a normal appearing proximal femur. This abnormal proximal femoral morphology leads to premature contact between the proximal femur and acetabulum through hip range of motion with resultant increase in shear forces seen by the labrum and acetabular cartilage.[17] While secondary causes of cam morphology have been well studied, the etiology of the idiopathic cam remains poorly understood.[18] It has been suggested that idiopathic cam morphology is multifactorial in nature and is influenced by many intrinsic and extrinsic factors including genetics, sporting activity, and hip morphology.

Genetics

Prior studies have suggested a role of genetic predisposition to the development of cam morphology. Pollard and colleagues evaluated 96 siblings of 64 patients who were treated for primary FAI and reported that the siblings of patients who had a cam deformity had a relative risk of 2.8 for having the same cam deformity, suggesting a genetic component to the etiology of cam impingement.[19] Faber and colleagues performed a genome-wide association study with alpha angle as a proxy to identify the genetic architecture of cam morphology use a UK Biobank study cohort of 44,214 participants.[20] They determined the heritability of alpha angle to be 10% and identified 8 independent genetic signals that were associated with alpha angle. Interestingly, their results identified a limited causal association between increasing alpha angle and the development of osteoarthritis. In contrast, there was a greater association between a genetic predisposition to osteoarthritis and an increased alpha angle.

Sporting Activity

Cam morphology has been reported to be highly prevalent in the adolescent athlete population. Young male athletes who participate in a range of sporting activities have been found to have a high rate of cam morphology with prevalence nearing 75%.[21–24] While challenging to elucidate, some evidence has suggested that participation in sports at a younger age predisposes patients to an increased risk of developing cam morphology.[25,26] Tak and colleagues retrospectively reviewed 63 soccer players for the presence of cam deformity on radiographs.[26] They reported that the prevalence of cam deformity was significantly higher in players who participated in higher frequency (≥4 times per week) soccer before the age of 12 years, which suggests a dose-dependent relationship between exposure to impingement related activities and development of cam morphology. Cam morphology in younger patients with high frequency-loading activity may be an adaptive response to a relative increase in shear stresses seen at the physis that subsequently results in physeal remodeling to improve stability and prevent slipped capital femoral epiphysis (SCFE).[18]

Hip Morphology

The abnormal shape of the proximal femur in cam morphology leads to FAI through varying degrees of hip motion. The position of motion at which cam impingement occurs is attributable to both the characteristics of the presenting cam morphology as well as patient-specific anatomic factors including but not limited to femoral version/torsion, acetabular overcoverage, acetabular version, and pelvic tilt.[2,27–29] An understanding of how each individual factor contributes to FAI can help to better understand why up to 14% to 23% of cam morphology can be asymptomatic in the general population.[30–32] In addition, knowledge of the influence of these anatomic factors can guide treatment of symptomatic cam morphology in FAI by understanding how each factor influences impingement patterns to ensure an adequate cam resection has been performed.

The relationship between femoral version/torsion and FAI has been well described. Both deformities result in alterations in proximal femoral anatomy that consequently leads to an increased risk of anterior impingement (femoral retroversion, femoral retrotorsion) or posterior impingement (femoral anteversion and femoral antetorsion) through hip motion.[27,33,34] Interestingly, impingement-free range of motion appears to be more heavily influenced by femoral version than the presence or absence of a cam lesion.[33,34] This highlights the complexity of treating patients with FAI and underlying proximal femoral rotational abnormalities. Fabricant and colleagues performed a prospective study evaluating the influence of femoral version on outcomes after arthroscopic management of FAI in 243 patients with an average of 21 months follow-up.[35] While they reported improvement in patient outcome measures for the entire cohort, a subanalysis of patients with femoral retroversion (<5° of femoral version) demonstrated less improvement compared to patients with normal version and femoral anteversion.

Acetabular sided abnormalities can also influence impingement-free motion in patients who present with associated cam morphology. Pincer impingement caused by excessive acetabular coverage (defined as lateral center edge angle > 40°) results in a more anterior impingement pattern with decreased hip flexion and internal rotation compared to normal acetabular morphology.[36] Decreased acetabular version creates both increased anterior coverage and decreased posterior coverage which subsequently produce a mixed impingement and instability presentation. Nearly a third of patients who present with symptomatic FAI have an underlying acetabular version abnormality.[29] It is important to identify patients with relative acetabular retroversion as they have been found to have both worse preoperative function and less improvement after hip arthroscopy for FAI.[37] Lastly, pelvic tilt can also influence impingement in patients with FAI as increased pelvic tilt creates functional acetabular overcoverage. Alterations in pelvic tilt can result in improvement in hip range of motion in the presence of cam morphology.[28,38]

Secondary Cam Morphology

Cam morphology can present as the sequelae of pre-existing hip pathology. Common causes of secondary cam morphology include SCFE, and Legg–Calve–Perthes disease (LCPD). The development of secondary cam morphology tends to be associated with symptomatic FAI, and the morphology and location of the cam is unique to the underlying pathology.

SCFE is the most common hip disorder in the adolescent population, occurring as frequently as 10.8 per 100,000 patients.[39] The postslip morphology after SCFE results in a posteriorly displaced and posteriorly tilted epiphysis and a resultant anterior and superior displacement of the metaphysis resulting in reduced femoral head–neck offset as well as loss of sphericity of the femoral head (**Fig. 1**A, B).[40] Additionally, shortening of the femoral neck can be observed which is associated with the amount of posterior displacement present.[41] In the post-SCFE deformity, the anterior metaphyseal bone results in cam impingement on the anterior acetabular rim.[39] Akiyama and colleagues evaluated the proximal femoral deformity seen in patients who underwent in situ pinning for stable SCFE at 63 months follow-up.[42] While some remodeling occurred that improved the abnormal alpha angle, the alpha angle and offset seen at final follow-up was still pathologic when compared to asymptomatic controls.

LCPD results in loss of sphericity of the pediatric femoral head secondary to osteonecrosis and subsequent collapse of the subchondral bone. Adaptive changes of the proximal femur to compensate for femoral head asphericity include a more prominent greater trochanter and a shortened femoral neck that is wider when compared to

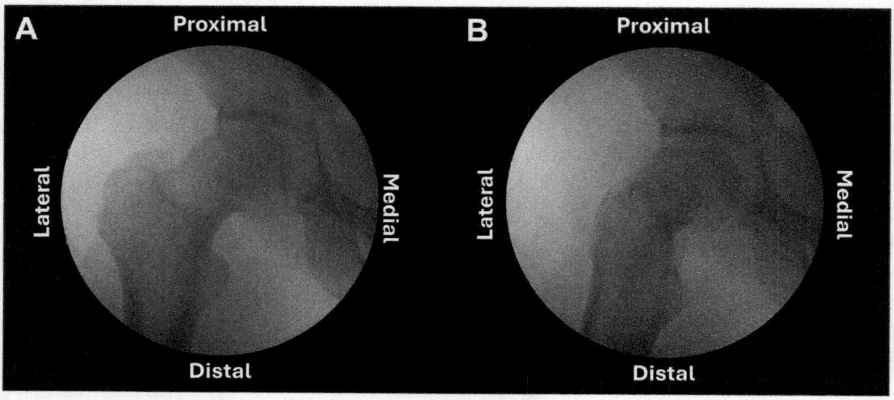

Fig. 1. Intraoperative fluoroscopy of a right hip with a post-SCFE deformity highlighting the posterior nature of the cam with the deformity that occurs at the level of the physis on the (*A*) anteroposterior and (*B*) extension with internal rotation views.

normal femoral neck.[41] Typical cam morphology in post-LCPD patients include prominent anterior and lateral cams that impinge on the acetabular rim.[43] While the more pressing manner in LCPD is worsening hip osteoarthritis, these patients develop symptomatic FAI before the onset of osteoarthritis, with up to 33% of individuals with LCPD presenting with symptomatic cam-type FAI.[44]

IMAGING MODALITIES

Diagnostic imaging plays a crucial role in the evaluation of patients who present with cam-type FAI. While history and physical provide useful information, the results of imaging studies can offer a more comprehensive understanding of the underlying pathology and provide insight to individualized patient-specific treatment.[12]

Radiographs

Radiographic evaluation is the preferred first-line imaging modality. While a substantial amount of information can be obtained from radiographs, it is important to understand that cam-type FAI is a 3-dimensional (3D) problem and can be difficult to assess with a 2-dimensional image. However, obtaining multiple radiographic views can provide critical information that can provide a more thorough understanding of the 3D pathology (**Fig. 2**A–C). For example, an anteroposterior (AP) pelvic radiograph can provide information on the lateral extent of the cam morphology on the proximal femur but may not provide adequate information on anterior or anterolateral (AL)-based cams. The cross-table lateral radiograph can assist with identification of more anteriorly based cam morphology and can identify femoral head–neck offset ratio difference between patients with and without symptomatic FAI.[45] The addition of 15° of internal rotation to the standard cross-table lateral can help improve inter- rater and intrarater reliability for assessment of cam morphology.[45] The modified Dunn view, which places the hip in either 90° or 45° of hip flexion and 20° of abduction with neutral rotation, was initially implemented for the assessment of femoral neck version in children.[46] The modified Dunn view places the hip in a position so that more AL-based cams can be well identified. Notably, the cross-table lateral with 15° of internal rotation and modified Dunn lateral have been reported to be the most sensitive radiographic views at detecting femoral head asphericity.[47] By understanding the anatomy of the AP,

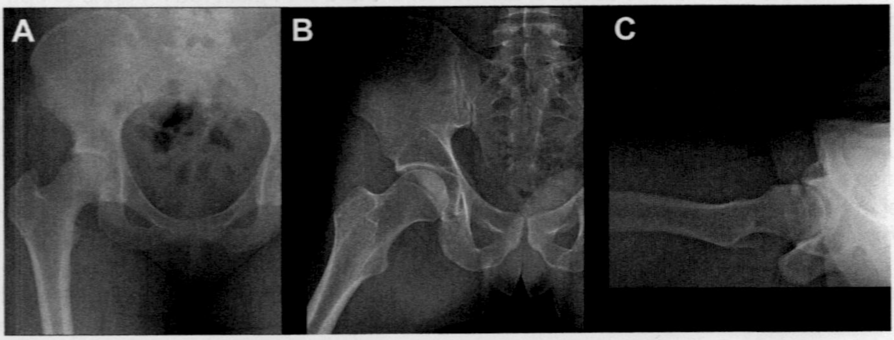

Fig. 2. Radiographic assessment of a right hip cam lesion cam lesion as seen on different views. (*A*) The anteroposterior pelvic radiograph provides visualization of a more posterolateral cam location. (*B*) The Dunn lateral radiograph positions the hip in a way that delivers a more AL cam into the plain of the radiograph for improved visualization. (*C*) The cross-table lateral provides visualization of a more anteriorly based cam lesion.

cross-table lateral, and modified Dunn radiograph, one can begin to conceptualize the 3D anatomy of the presenting cam morphology.

Advanced Imaging

Advanced imaging in the form of computed tomography (CT) scans and MRI can be useful in understanding cam morphology due to their ability to provide multiplanar images with high resolution. The alpha angle was initially established by Nötzil and colleagues with the use of an angled axial oblique MRI sequence to evaluate femoral head–neck junction abnormalities in patients with impingement.[48] Further work by Rakhra and colleagues identified that a radially oriented sequence can be more sensitive to detecting alpha angle when compared to an axial oblique oriented sequence.[49] One advantage MRI has over other imaging modalities is its ability to detect symptomatic soft-tissue cam impingement. Youngman and colleagues reviewed 332 patients who underwent MRI for symptomatic FAI to identify and characterize nonosseous cam impingement.[50] They found a 9% rate of soft-tissue impingement, with mean alpha angles greater on MRI than plain radiographs for patients with nonosseous cams. Findings consistent with soft-tissue cam impingement included a thickened perichondral ring, periosteal thickening, and cartilaginous epiphyseal extension.

CT scans can provide superior osseous detail when compared to MRI scans and are less dependent on patient position and sequence orientation.[51] CT scans can be particularly useful when assessing patients with abnormal cam morphology or secondary causes of FAI (such as SCFE or LCPD). The ability of CT scans to assess cam morphology can be even further enhanced through the use of 3D reconstructive models.[52,53] However, some studies suggest that the addition of 3D CT reconstruction may not provide any improved benefit in assessment of cam morphology when compared to plain radiographs. Cadet and colleagues performed a retrospective review of 8 patients who underwent surgery for FAI and had 4 observers (2 attending surgeons and 2 radiologists) assess preselected hip radiographs and 3D CT hip models.[54] They reported that alpha angles were significantly higher on plain radiographs compared to 3D CT reconstructions. Similarly, Smith and colleagues reported that the 45° Dunn lateral radiograph identified a higher alpha angle compared to MRI and CT.[55] While advanced imaging can play an important role in assessment of cam-type FAI, it is important to use as a tool in conjuncture with plain radiographs to optimize the assessment of cam morphology.

Ultrasonography

Ultrasonography (US) is less frequently used for the assessment of FAI but can be a useful adjunct as it is relatively inexpensive, quick, and can provide a real-time assessment of impingement through hip range of motion. While US has been found to be less effective at identifying labral pathology it can be useful in assessing cam-type impingement.[56,57] Lerch and colleagues used US to evaluate 40 patients with cam-type FAI as identified on oblique axial MRI.[57] They reported that there was no significant difference between alpha angle measured on MRI and US. Another advantage of US is its ability to provide a real-time dynamic assessment of the hip to determine impingement and instability patterns with substantial inter-rater agreement.[58,59] In this setting, US can be used to identify hip positioning and resultant impingement patterns that reproduce patient symptoms which can aid in planning a more patient-specific cam resection. However, while promising, the limitations in ultrasound assessment are dependent on user experience and proper training.[60]

Intraoperative Fluoroscopy

Arthroscopic femoral head–neck osteoplasty to treat cam-type FAI relies on both direct visualization via the arthroscopic assessment and indirect visualization with intraoperative fluoroscopic imaging.[61,62] Direct arthroscopic visualization combined with multiple fluoroscopic views in different positions allows for improved 3D conceptualization of the cam morphology to guide arthroscopic resection. Larson and Giveans discussed their fluoroscopic approach for intraoperative evaluation during hip arthroscopy for an "around-the-world" assessment of cam morphology.[62] This method begins with obtaining an AP pelvic radiograph in neutral abduction at 0 to 10° of hip flexion and maximal internal rotation, neutral rotation, maximal external rotation. They then proceed with flexion of the hip to 40° and additional radiographs are obtained with the hip in maximal internal rotation, neutral rotation, and maximal external rotation. The last fluoroscopic view obtained is a cross-table lateral. This method has been found to provide adequate assessment of cam deformities from 11:45 to 2:45 on the clock-face of the femoral head–neck junction.[63] Utilization of this *around-the-world* technique allows for a thorough intraoperative assessment of the presenting cam morphology to guide resection and ensure an adequate osteoplasty has been performed on multiple fluoroscopic views.

RESECTION TECHNIQUES AND OUTCOMES

Hip arthroscopy with cam resection for FAI is a technically demanding procedure with a steep learning curve.[64] The relatively high reported failure rate of 15.1% with revision rates ranging from 3.8% to 4.5% further highlight the difficulty of this procedure.[7,8,65] One of the most commonly reported causes of revision hip arthroscopy for cam-type FAI is inadequate resection.[8,9,65] A notable challenge in treating cam-type FAI with hip arthroscopy lies in the poor definition of what an adequate resection entails.

While alpha angle is commonly used in diagnosing cam-type FAI, its association with postoperative outcomes has been unreliable. Two retrospective studies by Lansdown and colleagues and Monohan and colleagues reported that postoperative alpha angle can be used as independent predictors of 2-year clinical outcomes and return to sport, respectively.[66,67] Conversely, Briggs and colleagues evaluated the correlation between alpha angle and 5-year outcomes in 230 patients after primary hip arthroscopy for cam-type FAI.[13] They reported no significant correlation between corrected alpha angle and patient reported outcomes. Similarly, Huang and colleagues retrospectively reviewed 159 patients with FAI to determine predictors of modified Harris Hip Score (mHHS) at 5-year follow-up.[14] In their study, age, preoperative mHHS, and postoperative Visual Analog Scale for pain scores were associated with postoperative mHHS. Notably, they identified almost no correlation between alpha angle and postoperative mHHS (Spearman correlation: 0.009). Lastly, Mansor and colleagues evaluated the effect of both over-resection (defined as resection over 5% of the diameter of the femoral head) and under-resection (defined as residual cam morphology with an alpha angle > 60°) on outcomes after hip arthroscopy.[10] Their results demonstrated that over-resection was associated with worse patient reported outcomes and an increased rate of conversion to total hip arthroplasty when compared to under-resection. Interestingly, there was limited difference in outcomes between the under-resection cohort and their neutral resection cohort, which continues to highlight limited correlation between alpha angle and postoperative outcomes. The results of these prior studies highlight the inadequacy of alpha angle as a radiographic measurement to guide intraoperative resection.

In addition to alpha angle, femoral head–neck offset is used in the preoperative assessment of FAI to determine the presence of pathologic cam morphology. Few studies have evaluated the influence of postoperative femoral head–neck offset on postoperative outcomes after hip arthroscopy. Haefeli and colleagues retrospectively reviewed 50 patients who underwent arthroscopic treatment for FAI and identified insufficient offset correction in the superior portion of the femoral neck to be a predictor for revision surgery.[15] In addition, Larson and colleagues retrospectively reviewed 79 patients who underwent revision arthroscopy for FAI at a mean 26 months follow-up.[16] In their study, improved femoral head–neck offset was a significant predictor for improved outcomes after revision hip arthroscopy. While these studies suggest that improvement in offset positively influences outcomes after hip arthroscopy, further work needs to be performed to better understand this relationship.

An ideal radiographic measurement to determine adequacy of cam resection would assess both femoral head sphericity (alpha angle) and femoral head–neck offset in a combined fashion to account for both parameters simultaneously. One novel radiographic measurement, the reflection index (RI) combines these 2 parameters to give a more comprehensive assessment of the cam resection (**Fig. 3**).[68] The RI uses the contour of the inferior femoral head–neck anatomy to establish the desired superior femoral head–neck anatomy, with an ideal RI representing symmetry between the 2 anatomic regions. The RI can be used for both preoperative assessment and intraoperative planning (**Fig. 4**A, B). Paliobeis and colleagues proposed utilization of this RI to assess postoperative outcomes after hip arthroscopy for FAI in a retrospective review of 63 hips.[68] They reported that a postoperative RI closer to 1 was an independent predictor of superior patient reported outcomes at 2 year follow-up, whereas

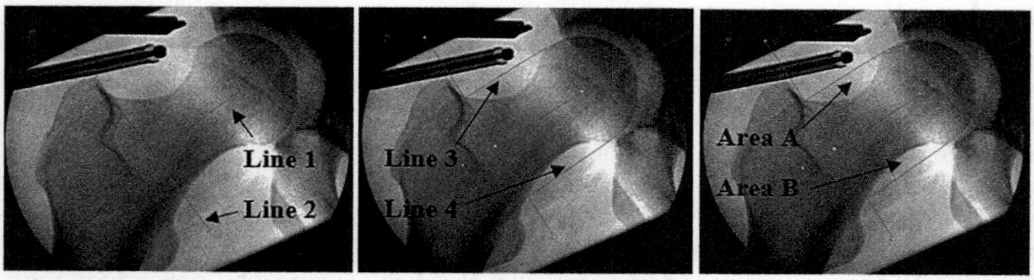

Fig. 3. RI measurement. Line 1 is drawn in line with the axis of the femoral neck from the center of the femoral head to the midpoint between the superior and inferior basicervical femoral neck. A perpendicular line (*line* 2) is then drawn at the level of the basicervical femoral neck. Two additional lines are drawn extending from the intersection of line 2 and the superior and inferior femoral neck to tangential points on the femoral head (*lines* 3 and 4). Line 3 begins at the superior aspect of the basicervical femoral neck just medial to the greater trochanter and extends medially to a tangential point on the superior aspect of the femoral head. Line 4 begins at the inferior aspect of the basicervical femoral neck just medial to the lesser trochanter and extends medially to a tangential point on the inferior aspect of the femoral head. The area between line 3 and a curvilinear line drawn along the superior femoral neck is defined as area A. The area between line 4 and another curvilinear line drawn along the inferior femoral neck is defined as area B. The RI is calculated by dividing area A by area B. (*From* Paliobeis AS, Strony JT, Ina JG, et al. Introducing the Reflection Index: A Novel Radiographic Assessment of Cam Morphology in Femoroacetabular Impingement and Predictor of Outcomes After Hip Arthroscopy With Minimum 2-Year Follow-up. Am J Sports Med 2025;53(9):2189–2197. https://doi.org/10.1177/03635465251346954.)

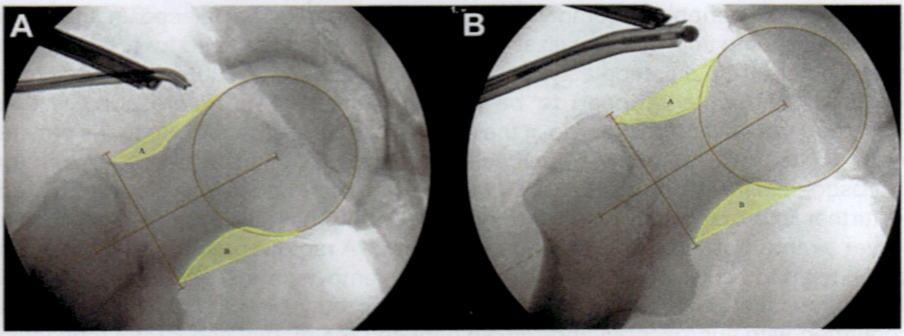

Fig. 4. Preoperative and postoperative RI examples. (*A*) Preresection intraoperative Dunn lateral fluoroscopic view. RI calculation: area A (3675)/area B (7930) = RI 0.463. (*B*) Postresection intraoperative Dunn lateral fluoroscopic view. RI calculation: area A (8391)/area B (7761) = RI 1.081. (*From* Paliobeis AS, Strony JT, Ina JG, et al. Introducing the Reflection Index: A Novel Radiographic Assessment of Cam Morphology in Femoroacetabular Impingement and Predictor of Outcomes After Hip Arthroscopy With Minimum 2-Year Follow-up. Am J Sports Med 2025;53(9):2189–2197. https://doi.org/10.1177/03635465251346954.)

alpha angle and head–neck offset ratio demonstrated no correlation with postoperative outcomes.

SURGICAL TECHNIQUE

Our preferred technique for cam resection is through an arthroscopic approach on a hip distraction table without a perineal post (**Fig. 5**). The arthroscopy is performed with a 3-portal technique use an AL portal, modified midanterior portal (MAP), and distal AL accessory portal. Intra-articular access is obtained under fluoroscopic guidance with the hip in traction. An interportal capsulotomy is performed between the AL portal and MAP. A diagnostic arthroscopy of the central compartment is then performed and all indicated procedures are performed. Once central compartment work is complete the hip is taken off traction and attention is then turned to the peripheral compartment.

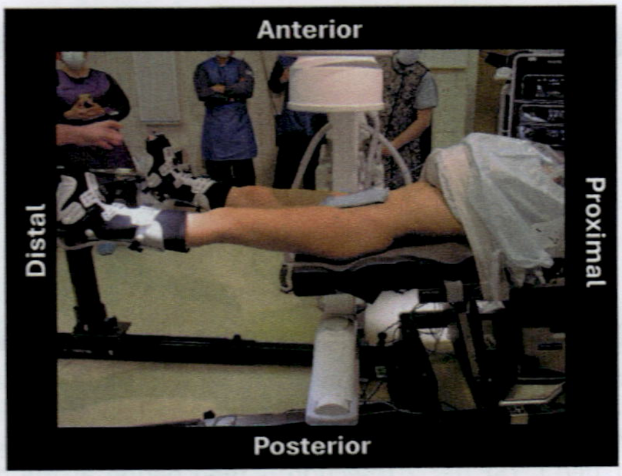

Fig. 5. The patient is positioned on a hip distraction table without the use of a perineal post. Fluoroscopy is positioned from the contralateral side and oriented perpendicular to the patient.

Once in the peripheral compartment, traction sutures are placed in the distal capsular leaflet to improve visualization (which precludes the need for a T-capsulotomy). To perform the osteoplasty, the reduced hip is flexed to 30° with neutral rotation, and the foot is dropped to be parallel with the bed. Fluoroscopy is then positioned from the opposite side of the operative table, perpendicular to the patient, with a 15° cranial tilt and 15° of rollback to produce a Dunn lateral image. With the arthroscope in the AL portal, the extent of the cam morphology can be appreciated. To further improve visualization the hip can be internally or externally rotated to deliver a more posterior or anterior cam into view. A radiofrequency ablation device is then used to define the zone of resection and remove periosteal tissue that would disrupt resection with the burr. Care is taken to stay distal to the physeal scar (confirmed with fluoroscopy) and remain between the medial and lateral retinacular vessels.

The goal of the femoral osteoplasty is to reestablish the proximal femoral head–neck offset and to recreate a spherical femoral head. Typically, we strive to mirror the offset and shape of the inferomedial side to restore the RI of the hip.[68] To do so, we use a 2-tiered resection method (**Fig. 6**A–C).[69] Viewing from the AL portal and working from the MAP, the proximal extent of the cam resection is defined by creating a trough roughly 8 mm (1.5 burr widths from the physeal scar using a 5.5 mm diameter burr) distal to the articular margin or physeal scar as identified on fluoroscopy. The location of this proximal tier (tier 1) also tends to be a few millimeters proximal to the lateral retinacular vessels which serve as an additional intraoperative landmark. The tier 1 resection is then performed to restore the native offset and establish the overall resection depth under fluoroscopic guidance. As the tier 1 resection is deepened the proximal head–neck junction is contoured to achieve the desired sphericity of the femoral head. Once the tier 1 resection is complete, a second parallel trough (tier 2) is created at the distal most extent of the planned resection of the cam and performed to the depth established at tier 1. The remainder of the cam between tier 1 and tier 2 is then resected to the set resection depth. The osteoplasty is continued between the established tiers on multiple fluoroscopic views as described by Larson and colleagues until the femoral offset and sphericity is restored in all planes.[62] With this 2-tiered technique we aim to avoid the often observed over-resected, proximally resected, and/or concave resection that

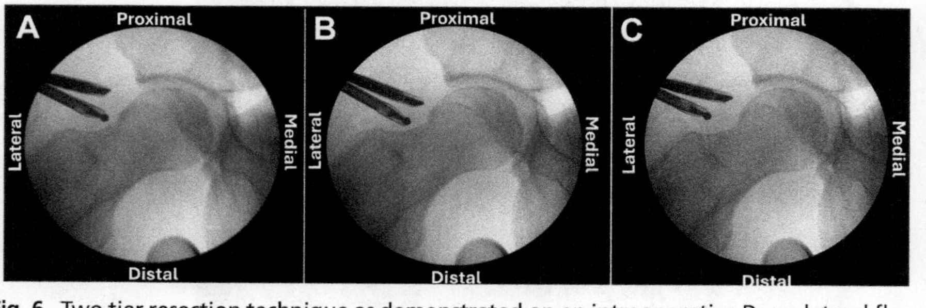

Fig. 6. Two tier resection technique as demonstrated on an intraoperative Dunn lateral fluoroscopic view of a right hip. (*A*) The tier 1 resection is started roughly 8 mm (1.5 burr widths with a 5.5 mm burr) distal to the physeal scar as identified on fluoroscopy. The resection depth is then set at tier 1. (*B*) Tier 2 resection is then begun at the distal aspect of the cam. The depth of resection of tier 2 is set to match the depth established at tier 1. The cam between tiers 1 and 2 is then resected to the set depth. (*C*) The proximal femoral head–neck junction is then contoured to recreate the femoral head sphericity.

prevents the restoration of native femoral head anatomy and disrupts the suction seal of the hip joint. Once the osteoplasty is complete final fluoroscopic views are obtained and the capsule is closed.

SUMMARY

FAI due to cam-type impingement can be challenging to address due to numerous etiologies and variation in hip anatomy that provide require a patient-specific approach to arthroscopic cam resection. While the history and physical play an important role in diagnosis of FAI, evaluation of imaging via radiographs, CT scan, MRI, and 3D reconstructions is vital in diagnosing and understanding the pathoanatomy. While there are established radiographic parameters for aiding in diagnosis of FAI (alpha angle and head–neck offset ratio), these parameters are poor predictors of patient reported outcomes after cam resection. Ultimately, the goal of the arthroscopic cam resection is to restore native femoral head sphericity and femoral head–neck offset ratio which can be reliably obtained use a 2-tier resection method, and measurements such as the RI that account for both of these factors may better predict postoperative outcomes.

CLINICS CARE POINTS

- Exposure to athletic high-frequency athletic activity at a younger age is associated with increased risk of development of cam morphology.[26]
- The 15° internally rotated cross-table lateral and modified Dunn lateral radiographs are the most sensitive radiographic views for assessing femoral head sphericity via alpha angle.[47]
- Inadequate resection of a cam lesion, particularly over-resection, can lead to worse outcomes and increased risk of conversion to total hip arthroplasty.[10]
- The reflection index is a novel radiographic measurement that can assist with intraoperative planning for arthroscopic cam resection has been found to better correlate with postoperative outcomes when compared to alpha angle and femoral head–neck offset ratio.[68]

DISCLOSURE

J. Ina and J. Kupriva have no conflicts of interest to disclose. Michael Salata has received consulting fees from Stryker.

REFERENCES

1. Hale RF, Melugin HP, Zhou J, et al. Incidence of femoroacetabular impingement and surgical management trends over time. Am J Sports Med 2021;49(1):35–41.
2. Beck M, Kalhor M, Leunig M, et al. Hip morphology influences the pattern of damage to the acetabular cartilage: femoroacetabular impingement as a cause of early osteoarthritis of the hip. J Bone Joint Surg Br 2005;87(7):1012–8.
3. Arciero E, Kakazu R, Garvin P, et al. Favorable patient-reported outcomes and high return to sport rates following hip arthroscopy in adolescent athletes: a systematic review. Arthroscopy 2022;38(9):2730–40.
4. Annin S, Lall AC, Yelton MJ, et al. Patient-reported outcomes in athletes following hip arthroscopy for femoroacetabular impingement with subanalysis on return to sport and performance level: a systematic review. Arthroscopy 2021;37(8): 2657–76.

5. Ramkumar PN, Olsen RJ, Shaikh HJF, et al. Modern hip arthroscopy for FAIS may delay the natural history of osteoarthritis in 25% of patients: a 12-Year Follow-up analysis. Am J Sports Med 2024;52(5):1137–43.
6. Adelstein JM, Sanghvi PA, Smith K, et al. Increased use of hip arthroscopy in the United States from 2015 to 2023 and projected growth through 2030. Arthroscopy 2025;41(10):3954–63.
7. Cevallos N, Soriano KKJ, Flores SE, et al. Hip arthroscopy volume and reoperations in a large cross-sectional population: high rate of subsequent revision hip arthroscopy in young patients and total hip arthroplasty in older patients. Arthroscopy 2021;37(12):3445–54.e1.
8. Degen RM, Pan TJ, Chang B, et al. Risk of failure of primary hip arthroscopy-a population-based study. J Hip Preserv Surg 2017;4(3):214–23.
9. Sardana V, Philippon MJ, de Sa D, et al. Revision hip arthroscopy indications and outcomes: a systematic review. Arthrosc J Arthrosc Relat Surg 2015;31(10):2047–55.
10. Mansor Y, Perets I, Close MR, et al. In search of the spherical femoroplasty: cam overresection leads to inferior functional scores before and after revision hip arthroscopic surgery. Am J Sports Med 2018;46(9):2061–71.
11. Mardones RM, Gonzalez C, Chen Q, et al. Surgical treatment of femoroacetabular impingement: evaluation of the effect of the size of the resection. J Bone Joint Surg Am 2005;87(2):273–9.
12. Ina J, Raji Y, Strony JT, et al. The role of imaging in femoroacetabular impingement: history, current practices, and future applications. JBJS Rev 2021;9(8). https://doi.org/10.2106/JBJS.RVW.21.00007.
13. Briggs KK, Soares E, Bhatia S, et al. Postoperative alpha angle not associated with patient-centered midterm outcomes following hip arthroscopy for FAI. Knee Surg Sports Traumatol Arthrosc 2019;27(10):3105–9.
14. Huang HJ, Dang HH, Mamtimin M, et al. Hip arthroscopy for femoroacetabular impingement syndrome shows good outcomes and low revision rates, with young age and low postoperative pain score predicting excellent 5-year outcomes. Arthroscopy 2023;39(2):285–92.
15. Haefeli PC, Albers CE, Steppacher SD, et al. What are the risk factors for revision surgery after hip arthroscopy for femoroacetabular impingement at 7-year followup? Clin Orthop 2017;475(4):1169–77.
16. Larson CM, Giveans MR, Samuelson KM, et al. Arthroscopic hip revision surgery for residual femoroacetabular impingement (FAI): surgical outcomes compared with a matched cohort after primary arthroscopic FAI correction. Am J Sports Med 2014;42(8):1785–90.
17. Ng KCG, Lamontagne M, Labrosse MR, et al. Hip joint stresses due to cam-type femoroacetabular impingement: a systematic review of finite element simulations. PLoS One 2016;11(1):e0147813.
18. Morris WZ, Li RT, Liu RW, et al. Origin of cam morphology in femoroacetabular impingement. Am J Sports Med 2017. https://doi.org/10.1177/0363546517697689.
19. Pollard TCB, Villar RN, Norton MR, et al. Genetic influences in the aetiology of femoroacetabular impingement: a sibling study. J Bone Joint Surg Br 2010;92(2):209–16.
20. Faber BG, Frysz M, Hartley AE, et al. A genome-wide association study meta-analysis of alpha angle suggests cam-type morphology may be a specific feature of hip osteoarthritis in older adults. Arthritis Rheumatol 2023;75(6):900–9.

21. Nepple JJ, Brophy RH, Matava MJ, et al. Radiographic findings of femoroacetabular impingement in national football league combine athletes undergoing radiographs for previous hip or groin pain. Arthroscopy 2012;28(10):1396–403.
22. Gerhardt MB, Romero AA, Silvers HJ, et al. The prevalence of radiographic hip abnormalities in elite soccer players. Am J Sports Med 2012;40(3):584–8.
23. Kapron AL, Anderson AE, Aoki SK, et al. Radiographic prevalence of femoroacetabular impingement in collegiate football players: AAOS exhibit selection. J Bone Jt Surg 2011;93(19):e111.
24. Larson CM, Sikka RS, Sardelli MC, et al. Increasing alpha angle is predictive of athletic-related "hip" and "groin" pain in collegiate National Football League prospects. Arthroscopy 2013;29(3):405–10.
25. Agricola R, Heijboer MP, Ginai AZ, et al. A cam deformity is gradually acquired during skeletal maturation in adolescent and young male soccer players: a prospective study with minimum 2-year follow-up. Am J Sports Med 2014;42(4):798–806.
26. Tak I, Weir A, Langhout R, et al. The relationship between the frequency of football practice during skeletal growth and the presence of a cam deformity in adult elite football players. Br J Sports Med 2015;49(9):630–4.
27. Tönnis D, Heinecke A. Acetabular and femoral anteversion: relationship with osteoarthritis of the hip. J Bone Joint Surg Am 1999;81(12):1747–70.
28. Kobayashi N, Higashihira S, Kitayama H, et al. Effect of decreasing the anterior pelvic tilt on range of motion in femoroacetabular impingement: a computer-simulation study. Orthop J Sports Med 2021;9(4):2325967121999464.
29. Arshad Z, Maughan HD, Sunil Kumar KH, et al. Over one third of patients with symptomatic femoroacetabular impingement display femoral or acetabular version abnormalities. Knee Surg Sports Traumatol Arthrosc 2021;29(9):2825–36.
30. Hack K, Di Primio G, Rakhra K, et al. Prevalence of cam-type femoroacetabular impingement morphology in asymptomatic volunteers. J Bone Joint Surg Am 2010;92(14):2436–44.
31. Frank JM, Harris JD, Erickson BJ, et al. Prevalence of femoroacetabular impingement imaging findings in asymptomatic volunteers: a systematic review. Arthroscopy 2015;31(6):1199–204.
32. Gosvig KK, Jacobsen S, Sonne-Holm S, et al. The prevalence of cam-type deformity of the hip joint: a survey of 4151 subjects of the copenhagen osteoarthritis study. Acta Radiol 2008;49(4):436–41.
33. Kraeutler MJ, Chadayammuri V, Garabekyan T, et al. Femoral version abnormalities significantly outweigh effect of cam impingement on hip internal rotation. J Bone Joint Surg Am 2018;100(3):205–10.
34. Ejnisman L, Philippon MJ, Lertwanich P, et al. Relationship between femoral anteversion and findings in hips with femoroacetabular impingement. Orthopedics 2013;36(3):e293–300.
35. Fabricant PD, Fields KG, Taylor SA, et al. The effect of femoral and acetabular version on clinical outcomes after arthroscopic femoroacetabular impingement surgery. J Bone Joint Surg Am 2015;97(7):537–43.
36. Kubiak-Langer M, Tannast M, Murphy SB, et al. Range of motion in anterior femoroacetabular impingement. Clin Orthop 2007;458:117–24.
37. Larson JH, Allahabadi S, Kaplan D, et al. Exploring the relationship between combined, acetabular, and femoral version on postoperative outcomes 2 years after hip arthroscopy for femoroacetabular impingement syndrome. Am J Sports Med 2025;53(2):269–80.

38. Swärd Aminoff A, Agnvall C, Todd C, et al. The effect of pelvic tilt and cam on hip range of motion in young elite skiers and nonathletes. Open Access J Sports Med 2018;9:147–56.
39. Novais EN, Millis MB. Slipped capital femoral epiphysis: prevalence, pathogenesis, and natural history. Clin Orthop 2012;470(12):3432–8.
40. Goodman DA, Feighan JE, Smith AD, et al. Subclinical slipped capital femoral epiphysis. Relationship to osteoarthrosis of the hip. J Bone Joint Surg Am 1997;79(10):1489–97.
41. Chan EF, Farnsworth CL, Koziol JA, et al. Statistical shape modeling of proximal femoral shape deformities in legg-calvé-perthes disease and slipped capital femoral epiphysis. Osteoarthr Cartil 2013;21(3):443–9.
42. Akiyama M, Nakashima Y, Kitano T, et al. Remodelling of femoral head-neck junction in slipped capital femoral epiphysis: a multicentre study. Int Orthop 2013;37-(12):2331–6.
43. Snow SW, Keret D, Scarangella S, et al. Anterior impingement of the femoral head: a late phenomenon of Legg-Calvé-Perthes' disease. J Pediatr Orthop 1993;13(3):286–9.
44. Accadbled F, Pailhé R, Launay F, et al. "Femoroacetabular impingement". Legg-Calve-perthes disease: from childhood to adulthood. Orthop Traumatol Surg Res 2014;100(6):647–9.
45. Eijer H, Leunig M, Mahomed MN, et al. Cross-table lateral radiographs for screening of anterior femoral head-neck offset in patients with femoro-acetabular impingement. HIP Int 2001;11(1):37–41.
46. Dunn DM. Anteversion of the neck of the femur; a method of measurement. J Bone Joint Surg Br 1952;34-B(2):181–6.
47. Meyer DC, Beck M, Ellis T, et al. Comparison of six radiographic projections to assess femoral head/neck asphericity. Clin Orthop 2006;445:181–5.
48. Nötzli HP, Wyss TF, Stoecklin CH, et al. The contour of the femoral head-neck junction as a predictor for the risk of anterior impingement. J Bone Joint Surg Br 2002;84-B(4):556–60.
49. Rakhra KS, Sheikh AM, Allen D, et al. Comparison of MRI alpha angle measurement planes in femoroacetabular impingement. Clin Orthop 2009;467(3):660–5.
50. Youngman TR, Johnson BL, Morris WZ, et al. Soft tissue cam impingement in adolescents: MRI reveals impingement lesions underappreciated on radiographs. Am J Sports Med 2023;51(14):3749–55.
51. Ekhtiari S, Fairhurst O, Mainwaring L, et al. The alpha angle. J Bone Jt Surg 2024;106(20):1910.
52. Beaulé PE, Zaragoza E, Motamedi K, et al. Three-dimensional computed tomography of the hip in the assessment of femoroacetabular impingement. J Orthop Res 2005;23(6):1286–92.
53. Abel MF, Sutherland DH, Wenger DR, et al. Evaluation of CT scans and 3-D reformatted images for quantitative assessment of the hip. J Pediatr Orthop 1994;14(1):48–53.
54. Cadet ER, Babatunde OM, Gorroochurn P, et al. Inter- and intra-observer agreement of femoroacetabular impingement (FAI) parameters comparing plain radiographs and advanced, 3D computed tomographic (CT)-generated hip models in a surgical patient cohort. Knee Surg Sports Traumatol Arthrosc 2016;24(7):2324–31.
55. Smith KM, Gerrie BJ, McCulloch PC, et al. Comparison of MRI, CT, Dunn 45° and Dunn 90° alpha angle measurements in femoroacetabular impingement. Hip Int 2018;28(4):450–5.

56. Troelsen A, Jacobsen S, Bolvig L, et al. Ultrasound versus magnetic resonance arthrography in acetabular labral tear diagnostics: a prospective comparison in 20 dysplastic hips. Acta Radiol Stockh Swed 1987 2007;48(9):1004–10.
57. Lerch S, Kasperczyk A, Warnecke J, et al. Evaluation of Cam-type femoroacetabular impingement by ultrasound. Int Orthop 2013;37(5):783–8.
58. Rosenberg SI, Soliman SB, Gornitzky AL, et al. Ultrasound evaluation of the hip. Curr Rev Musculoskelet Med 2024;17(12):548–58.
59. Sahr ME, Endo Y, Sink EL, et al. Dynamic ultrasound assessment of hip instability and anterior and posterior hip impingement. Skelet Radiol 2023;52(7):1385–93.
60. Mullaney PJ. Qualitative ultrasound training: defining the learning curve. Clin Radiol 2019;74(4). https://doi.org/10.1016/j.crad.2018.12.018. 327.e7-327.e19.
61. Byrd JWT, Jones KS. Arthroscopic femoroplasty in the management of cam-type femoroacetabular impingement. Clin Orthop 2009;467(3):739–46.
62. Larson CM, Giveans MR. Arthroscopic management of femoroacetabular impingement: early outcomes measures. Arthroscopy 2008;24(5):540–6.
63. Ross JR, Bedi A, Stone RM, et al. Intraoperative fluoroscopic imaging to treat cam deformities: correlation with 3-Dimensional computed tomography. Am J Sports Med 2014;42(6):1370–6.
64. Dumont GD, Cohn RM, Gross MM, et al. The learning curve in hip arthroscopy: effect on surgical times in a single-surgeon cohort. Arthroscopy 2020;36(5): 1293–8.
65. Malviya A, Raza A, Jameson S, et al. Complications and survival analyses of hip arthroscopies performed in the national health service in England: a review of 6,395 cases. Arthroscopy 2015;31(5):836–42.
66. Lansdown DA, Kunze K, Ukwuani G, et al. The importance of comprehensive cam correction: radiographic parameters are predictive of patient-reported outcome measures at 2 years after hip arthroscopy. Am J Sports Med 2018; 46(9):2072–8.
67. Monahan PF, Jimenez AE, Owens JS, et al. Postoperative alpha angle is predictive of return to sport in athletes undergoing hip arthroscopy for femoroacetabular impingement. Arthroscopy 2022;38(4):1204–14.
68. Paliobeis AS, Strony JT, Ina JG, et al. Introducing the reflection index: a novel radiographic assessment of cam morphology in femoroacetabular impingement and predictor of outcomes after hip arthroscopy with minimum 2-Year Follow-up. Am J Sports Med 2025;53(9):2189–97.
69. Haase L, Secretov E, Nelson G, et al. Two-tiered resection of cam lesions in hip femoroacetabular impingement: optimizing femoral head sphericity. Arthrosc Tech 2022;11(7):e1311–6.

Hip Arthroscopy in Dysplasia: Addressing Anatomy and Setting Yourself up for Periacetabular Osteotomy Success

Brenden Ronna, MD*, Alexandria Chrumka, MD,
Andrea Spiker, MD

KEYWORDS

• Hip arthroscopy • Periacetabular osteotomy • PAO • Hip preservation
• Combined hip arthroscopy and PAO

KEY POINTS

- Combined hip arthroscopy and periacetabular osteotomy (PAO) can be used to both address the intraarticular pathology associated with hip dysplasia as well as correct the dysplastic anatomy.
- Combining hip arthroscopy with a PAO is associated in improved outcomes in patients with dysplasia and concomitant intra-articular or extra-articular pathology.
- Modifications to the arthroscopic proceduring including illiocapsularis dissection from the underlying capsule after capsular closure can aid in beginning the dissection for PAO.

Video content accompanies this article at http://www.sportsmed.theclinics.com.

BACKGROUND

Hip arthroscopy continues to be a growing area of research and clinical practice within orthopedic sports medicine. The number of hip arthroscopy cases performed has increased exponentially over the past 2 decades.[1] While hip arthroscopy for femoroacetabular impingement as well as labral and intra-articular pathology has shown excellent outcomes,[2–4] one area of continued debate and exploration is hip arthroscopy in the dysplastic and borderline dysplastic patient.

Department of Orthopedic Surgery, University of Wisconsin-Madison, 600 Highland Avenue, Madison, WI 53705, USA
* Coresponding author.
E-mail address: Brenden.ronna@gmail.com

Clin Sports Med 45 (2026) 663–674
https://doi.org/10.1016/j.csm.2026.03.008 sportsmed.theclinics.com

Abbreviations	
DALA	distal anterolateral accessory
FEAR	Femoro-Epiphyseal Acetabular Roof
IC	iliocapsularis
LCEA	lateral center edge angle
MR	magnetic resonance
PAO	periacetabular osteotomy
PROMs	patient reported outcome measures
RFA	radiofrequency ablation
THA	total hip arthroplasty

Hip dysplasia is defined as an acetabulum, which has a decreased depth as well as deficiency in shape and/or orientation leading to an overall undercoverage of the femoral head, smaller contact area between the femoral head and acetabulum as well as a lateralized hip center of rotation.[5] Hip dysplasia is a common cause of hip pain and dysfunction as well as a leading cause of hip osteoarthritis.[6–8] The prevalence of hip dysplasia in patients presenting with hip pain has been reported around 8% to 9%, and dysplasia is reported to be present in 20% to 40% of patients with hip osteoarthritis.[1] Continued research has allowed us a better understanding of the nuances of hip dysplasia diagnosis, which is important as missed hip dysplasia or instability is a recognized cause of hip arthroscopy failure. Understanding not only how to diagnose dysplasia, but how to modify surgical techniques in the setting of borderline dysplasia, can help us optimize our surgical outcomes.

The radiographic definition of hip dysplasia is based on the lateral center edge angle (LCEA). Patients with an LCEA less than 25° are defined as having dysplasia, or acetabular undercoverage, while those greater than 25° are defined as having normal acetabular coverage. Borderline hip dysplasia is typically defined as 18 to 25° (or classified 20–25° in some publications).[9,10] Other radiographic measurements can be used to augment the LCEA, such as the Femoro-Epiphyseal Acetabular Roof (FEAR) index. It is calculated by measuring the angle between a line along the acetabular sourcil and a line along the physeal scar of the femoral head. A FEAR index greater than 5° is associated with dysplasia.[11]

The treatment of hip dysplasia is based on multiple factors including the degree of dysplasia, patient age, concomitant pathology (ie, labral tears), soft tissue integrity, and presence or absence of osteoarthritic changes. The Bernese periacetabular osteotomy (PAO) has evolved as the standard of care to correct symptomatic dysplasia since its description over 3 decades ago.[12] PAO has demonstrated long term hip survivorship between 74% and 92% over 10 years.[13–15] Additionally, surgical correction of hip dysplasia with PAO has been shown to significantly improve patient reported outcome measures (PROMs).[16,17] However, as described by Nepple and colleagues, 11% of patients continue to have hip symptoms post-PAO.[18] As many as 60% to 85% of patients with symptomatic hip dysplasia have been described to have concomitant chondral and or labral pathology.[19–21] There is also a relatively high prevalence of cam deformity in dysplastic patients.[22] As a result, there is growing interest and advocacy of combining a PAO with hip arthroscopy to address the intra-articular and extra-articular pathology to improve clinical outcomes,[23–25] Combined hip arthroscopy with PAO is emerging as a controversial topic given a recent randomized control study investigating the utility of adding hip arthroscopy to PAO, which suggested no additional improvement in outcomes when adding a hip arthroscopy.[26] While the mainstay indication of PAO is in fact hip dysplasia, it is also important to note that the PAO can also be used when traditional hip dysplasia is not present, such as in cases of acetabular retroversion.[27]

The purpose of this review is to summarize the literature of hip arthroscopy and combined PAO in the treatment of hip dysplasia and to detail the technical aspects of combined arthroscopy to assist in PAO dissection and a successful procedure.

COMBINED PERIACETABULAR OSTEOTOMY AND HIP ARTHROSCOPY FOR SYMPTOMATIC HIP DYSPLASIA

Patients with symptomatic hip dysplasia have a high prevalence of intraarticular pathology, with one series demonstrating chondral or labral damage in up to 78% in prearthritic dysplastic hips (female adolescents aged 12–19).[28] Additionally, CAM lesions have been reported in one study to be as high as 22% in Tönnis grade 0 or 1 dysplastic hips and as high as 50% in Tönnis grade 2.[22] However it is important to note that asymptomatic CAM lesions have also been demonstrated to be 37% to 55% in athletes and around 23% in the general population (Frank and colleagues, 2015).These concomitant intraarticular pathologies have demonstrated excellent outcomes when treated with hip arthroscopy in the setting of hip dysplasia.[2–4]

The outcomes of combined PAO and hip arthroscopy have been published in several recent studies, demonstrating favorable outcomes of the combined procedures.[29] A series of 16 patients (average age 23.5) undergoing PAO with combined hip arthroscopy demonstrated significant improvement in modified harris hip score, nonarthritic hip score, Hip Outcome Score-Sports-Specific Subscale and visual analog pain scale (VAS) pain score ($P<.007$) at 5 years with no conversion to total hip arthroplasty (THA).[30] Another series in 29 athletes (mean age 26.0 years) undergoing PAO and arthroscopy for dysplasia with a concomitant CAM lesion demonstrated significant improvement in patient reported outcomes as well as a return to sport rate of 81.8% at 2 year follow-up.[31] Additionally, recent systematic reviews have discussed significant improvements in PROMs with combined PAO and hip arthroscopy.[32,33]

While many studies show significant improvement in PROMs after combined hip arthroscopy and PAO, other studies have failed to show a difference between PAO alone versus PAO with hip arthroscopy with regards to PROMs.[26,33] In their randomized controlled study of 192 patients, PAO alone PAO plus hip arthroscopy, Beaule demonstrated that patients in both groups had significant improvement in functional outcomes at 1 year.[26] At the 1 year mark, 4 patients in the PAO alone group underwent subsequent hip arthroscopy for persistent symptoms compared to 1 patient in the PAO plus hip arthroscopy cohort (Beaule, 2024). This randomized study demonstrated noninferiority of adding hip arthroscopy to PAO; however approximately 51% of the *PAO* group had additional intra-articular or extra-articular work performed (cam decompression (35%) or subspine decompression [16%]), which could add bias to their findings.[26]

HIP ARTHROSCOPY AFTER PERIACETABULAR OSTEOTOMY IN SYMPTOMATIC HIP DYSPLASIA

Another important question regarding the combination of hip arthroscopy and PAO relates to timing of the 2 procedures. Hip arthroscopy, when performed as a second, revision, procedure after PAO, has not demonstrated improved outcomes. In one retrospective study of 202 patients undergoing PAO, 15 patients required hip arthroscopy at a mean time of 3.9 years (0.3–10.3 years) after PAO. These hips had Tönnis 0 (n = 12) or Tönnis 1 (n = 3) changes. All hips had a labral tear and 9/15 that demonstrated chondral damage greater than Beck 4. 4/15 were converted to a THA at a mean of 1.8 years after arthroscopy.[34] There were also no significant improvements in PROMs. It should be noted that 8/15 labral tears were treated with debridement alone and those patients converted to a THA were older (P = .01) and had lower post-PAO LCEA (27° in patients converted to THA compared to 40° in patients not requiring THA) (P = .01).[34]

COMBINED HIP ARTHROSCOPY AND PERIACETABULAR OSTEOTOMY TECHNIQUE

Preoperative Workup and Indications

In the authors' practice, patients are indicated for PAO if they are diagnosed with symptomatic hip dysplasia. Preoperative workup includes standard radiographs (standing anteroposterior pelvis, false profile, 45° Dunn lateraland Von Rosen views), magnetic resonance (MR) imaging and a low radiation dose 3-dimentianal computed tomography scan per our hip-preservation reconstruction protocols.[35] The patient is indicated for a combined (concomitant) hip arthroscopy and PAO if the patient is found to have hip dysplasia with preoperative MRI demonstrating labral or other intra-articular pathology, which is found to be clinically symptomatic on history and clinical examination.[35]

Hip Arthroscopy Immediately Preceding Periacetabular Osteotomy

It is the authors' preference to perform hip arthroscopy immediately before PAO as the arthroscopic portion of the case not only addresses intra-articular pathology (including labral tears and unstable cartilage), but may also aid in dissection for the PAO portion of the case. In the authors' experience, arthroscopic cam decompression (femoral osteochondroplasty) is more efficient, comprehensive and accurate than open, and capsular repair is also more expeditiously performed arthroscopically compared to open. Using the same preparation and drape, we proceed with the PAO immediately after the hip arthroscopy. In cases where arthroscopy and PAO cannot be immediately performed together in one anesthetic event, we prefer to perform the 2 procedures in sequence as soon as possible. **Fig. 1** demonstrates our preferred sterile back table set up.

The patient is placed supine on the traction table, with our preference being postless traction. The table should also be radiolucent as the use of a nonradiolucent table requires the patient to be transferred from the traction table to a second radiolucent table (**Fig. 2**). Several modifications are made to the hip arthroscopy technique when arthroscopy is immediately preceding a PAO. As described in Spiker and colleagues's reports[35,36]: Suggested modifications include minimizing capsule disruption, performing labral repair or reconstruction as appropriate, performing arthroscopic cam and/or subspine decompression as necessary, and completing an arthroscopic capsular closure. A complete list of suggested modifications is listed in **Box 1**.

During hip arthroscopy, a small interportal capsulotomy is created and chondral and labral pathology noted and addressed. If a Cam lesion is present, it can be addressed open, however our preference is to address the deformity arthroscopically. The capsule will then be fully repaired arthroscopically (**Fig. 3**). A modification when performed immediately preceding PAO is the dissection of the iliocapsularis (IC) off of the anterior hip capsule, beginning laterally, and proceeding until the iliopsoas tendon sheath is reached (**Fig. 4**). Capsular repair before this step will restore tension to the hip capsule and aid in iliocapsularis elevation, which is performed with the radiofrequency ablation device. Care is taken to ensure the dissection stays superficial to the capsule to thus maintain capsular integrity. This dissection is carried medially until the psoas bursa is identified. The IC dissection is continued proximally where the IC is dissected off the direct head of the rectus tendon, with safe visualization being crucial (**Fig. 5** and Video 1). The remaining fibers of the IC attached to the rectus will be

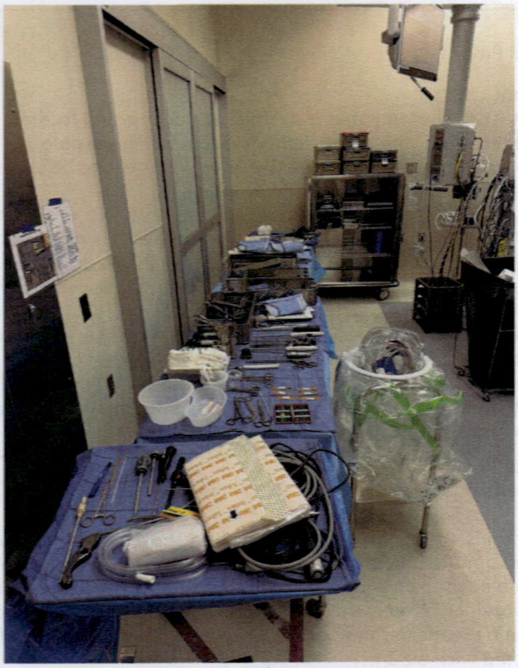

Fig. 1. Demonstration of the set up on the back table for combined hip arthroscopy + PAO.

dissected from the medial direct head of the rectus tendon during the PAO exposure (Video 1).

At the conclusion of hip arthroscopy, portals are completely closed with interrupted nylon suture.

Transition to Periacetabular Osteotomy Positioning

For the PAO portion of the case, the same, postless radiolucent traction table is used. The traction boots are removed, an extension table is placed, and the hip arthroscopy

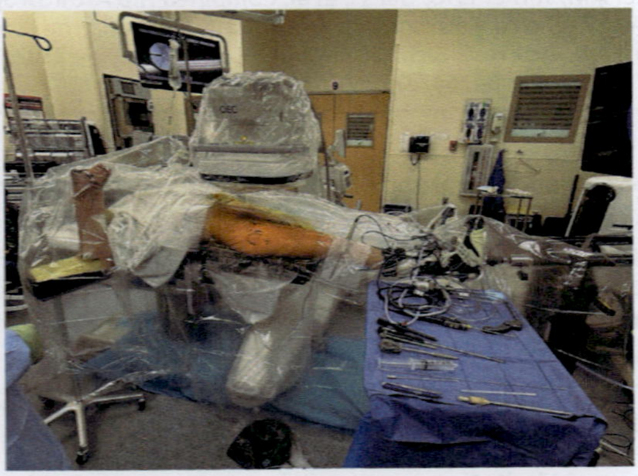

Fig. 2. Demonstrates the set up for the hip arthroscopy portion of the case with the legs in traction, use of the shower curtain drape and the C-Arm coming in from the opposite side relatively to the operative site.

Box 1
Technical Pearls and Pitfalls

Central Compartment

Perform interportal capsulotomy that is as small as possible and located laterally (staying lateral to the direct head of the rectus femoris origin when possible).

Two portals can be used (particularly if the CAM does not need to be addressed or if it will be addressed with open capsulotomy after the PAO).

If using 2 portals, they must provide an adequate trajectory for suture anchor placement. distal anterolateral accessory (DALA) portal can be created if a more distal-to-proximal trajectory is needed in labral repair, as is often the case in the dysplastic acetabulum. The DALA is the portal through, which we prefer instrumenting through during arthroscopic CAM resection.

In the setting of labral repair, the use of simple suture repair versus mattress suture repair depends on the quality and morphology of the labral tissue.

Perform careful evaluation of the articular cartilage surfaces. Should the chondral wear be more significant than estimated on preoperative imaging, this might be a decision point on whether or not performing the PAO is indicated.

Peripheral Compartment

Traction is removed and the hip is flexed to 30° to 45°. Tension on the traction boots is released.

If no significant cam is present, or if the cam will be addressed through an open approach after the PAO, additional arthroscopic work in the peripheral compartment is not necessary. Should a cam lesion need to be addressed arthroscopically, visualization of the femoral head/neck junction is obtained. Placement of suspension sutures in the distal capsule versus a T-capsulotomy can be made with radiofrequency ablation (RFA) device if needed. The cam can then be resected with a burr.

The interportal capsulotomy can then be closed arthroscopically or via open repair after the PAO is completed. It is the authors' preference to close the T-capsulotomy and interportal capsulotomies arthroscopically to restore the tension to the hip capsule before performing further dissection in preparation for the PAO.

Dissection of the iliocapsularis off of the hip capsule can then be performed with a radiofrequency ablation device with care taken to minimize damage to the capsule as well as the iliocapsularis. Dissection is carried medially off of the capsule until the psoas bursa has been identified.

Proximally, the iliocapsularis can be dissected off of the medial edge of the direct head of the rectus tendon as far as can be safely visualized, with the remaining fibers of the iliocapsularis being dissected from the medial rectus tendon during open PAO approach.

Adapted from Spiker AM, Turner EHG, Gans I, et al. Combined Hip Arthroscopy and Periacetabular Osteotomy (PAO): Technical Focus on Arthroscopically Elevating the Iliocapsularis and Performing the Open PAO. Arthrosc Tech. 2021 Sep 21;10(10):e2293–e2302. https://doi.org/10.1016/j.eats.2021.07.004. PMID: 34754737; PMCID: PMC8556612.

portals are covered. An additional shower curtain drape is placed on the other side of table. A triangle is placed under the knee (nonsterile) as needed (**Fig. 6**).

If hip arthroscopy was performed on a nonradiolucent table, the patient must be transferred to a radiolucent table for the PAO portion. The nonoperative leg is well padded and secured. The patient is reprepped and redraped if transfer to a radiolucent table is performed.

Fig. 7 demonstrates the preferred incisions and anatomic markings for both the hip arthroscopy and the PAO.

Advantages, Risks, and Limitations

There are several practical advantages to combining hip arthroscopy with PAO such as allowing all intra-articular pathology to be addressed at the same surgical setting as the

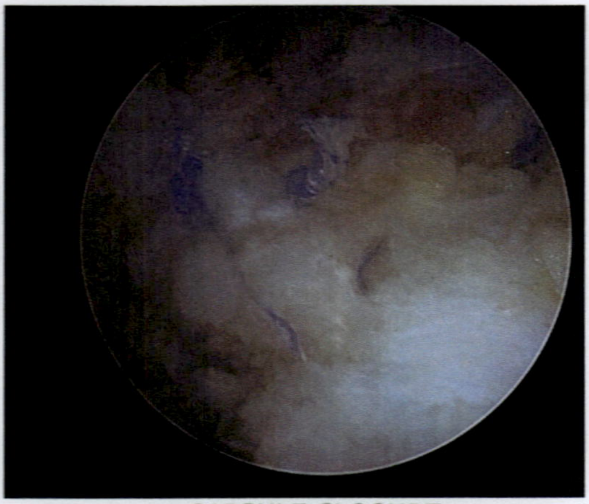

Fig. 3. Capsule closure after intraarticular labral work and CAM decompression but before iliocapsularis dissection.

acetabular reorientation. Additionally, the IC muscle may be dissected off of the capsule which allows for efficient dissection, which would otherwise be performed open.

However, combining these procedures is not without risks or limitations. First, hip arthroscopy may result in fluid extravasation. The authors find that the fluid dissection results in hydrodissection of the tissue planes, which can actually be advantageous. If the postless radiolucent table is not available, the patient must be transferred to a second table, which is radiolucent after completion of the hip arthroscopy. Additionally, the ability to perform these procedures efficiently and safely requires a team of surgeons or surgeon who can perform both the hip arthroscopy and open PAO. If more than one surgeon are involved, logistics of scheduling the individual surgeries can add complexity to performing a combined case.

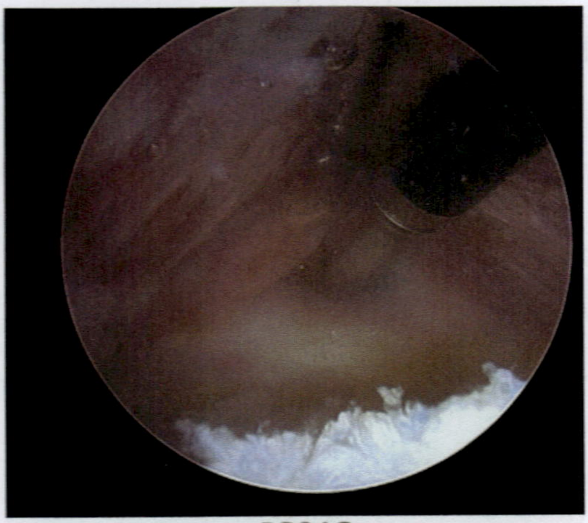

Fig. 4. IC dissection carried medially over to the Psoas Bursa. Psoas tendon visualized inferior to the RFA device.

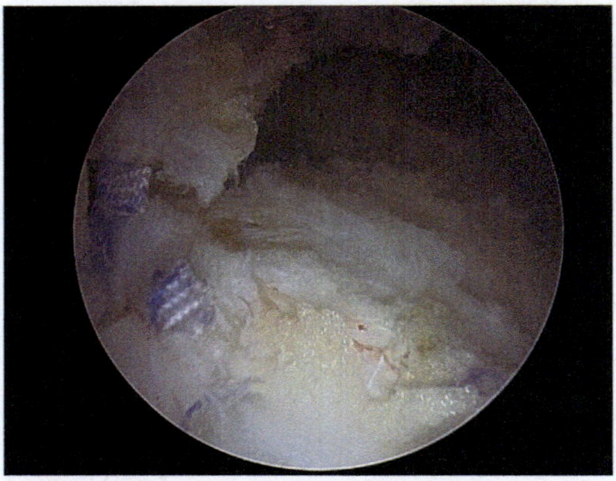

Fig. 5. Complete IC dissection off of the capsule, with the closed capsule in the foreground.

DISCUSSION

Hip dysplasia is a common condition, which can lead to hip pain and is a precursor for hip osteoarthritis.[1,6–8] The recognition of dysplasia in patients with hip pain is increasing with better diagnostic tools and heightened awareness. Symptomatic hip dysplasia is best addressed with the Bernese periacetabular osteotomy, which has demonstrated improved functional, and patient reported outcomes as well as hip survivability.[13–17] However, there are several dysplastic patients who also present with symptomatic intra-articular or extra-articular hip pathology such as labral tears, chondral lesions, CAM lesions and/or subspine impingement.[19,21–23] As such, there are dysplastic patients who undergo PAO who then must subsequently undergo hip arthroscopy for these ongoing, unaddressed conditions.[34] Performing concomitant hip arthroscopy with PAO is a solution to address both intra-articular pathology and dysplasia in one surgical setting.

Hip arthroscopy is a growing field and has demonstrated excellent outcomes for both intra-and extra-articular hip pathologies.[2–4] Likewise, PAO has demonstrated excellent long-term outcomes in isolation.[13–15] A current and ongoing question is whether the combination of hip arthroscopy and PAO for the symptomatic hip

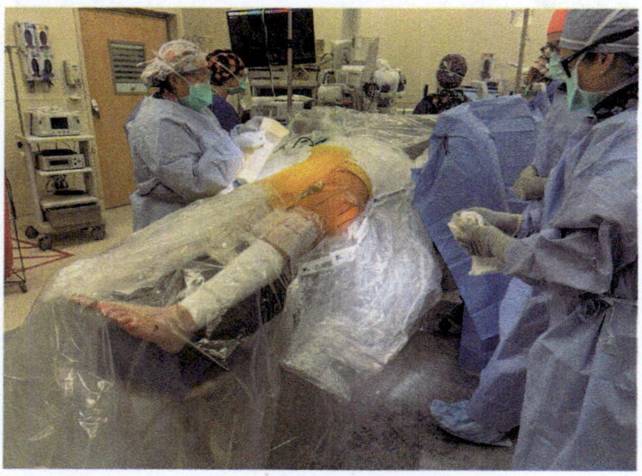

Fig. 6. The patient is removed from traction and now the operative site is reprepped and draped without a position change for the PAO portion of the case.

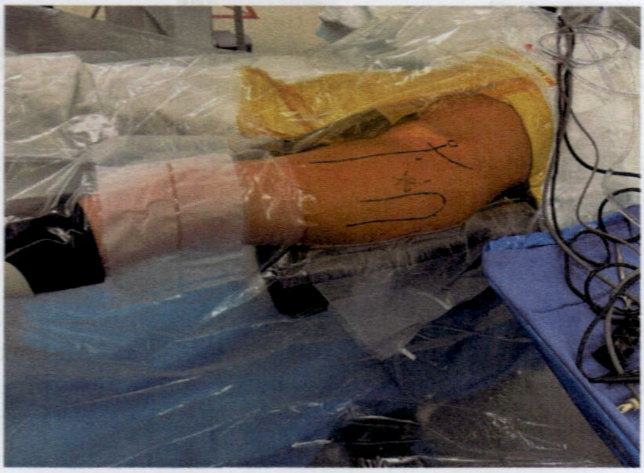

Fig. 7. Demonstration of the anatomic markings used in combined hip arthroscopy including the greater trochanter, lateral femur, and the ASIS. Midanterior and anterolateral arthroscopy portals are drawn as well as the incision for the PAO proximally.

dysplasia patient with concomitant labral, chondral or CAM pathology is of benefit to our patients. Our indication for combined procedures is a patient who has failed conservative management, who also demonstrates symptomatic labral, chondral or CAM pathology in history, clinical examination and imaging (ie, X-ray [XR] and MR).

Hip arthroscopy at the time of PAO has demonstrated significant improvement in patient reported and functional outcomes[30,31](Maldonado 2019; Jimenez 2022) with a return to sport rate of 81.8% at 2 years in one series.[31] The ability to visualize, diagnose and treat intra-articular and extra-articular pathology is thought to increase satisfaction and functional outcomes after the PAO procedure (Sabbag and colleagues, 2019). While the combined procedure does have risks and limitations such as fluid extravasation, potential need for a second table and requirement for a team and surgeon to be proficient in both procedures, the procedure has been demonstrated to be safe. One retrospective review demonstrated a complication rate of combined hip arthroscopy and PAO of 3%, similar to previously published PAO alone complications.[37]

While these studies have demonstrated the safety and efficacy of combined hip arthroscopy and PAO, several other studies have demonstrated good outcomes in PAO alone or no difference in PAO alone compared to hip arthroscopy plus PAO. In a recent randomized controlled showed that patients in the PAO alone and PAO + Hip arthroscopy cohorts both demonstrated improvements in functional scores at 12 months. However, the 1 year follow-up is an acknowledged limitation and further follow-up will be required to evaluate long term differences between groups.[26] In their analysis, they noted no difference in patient reported outcome measures at 1 year between PAO versus PAO + hip arthroscopy with labral management. Additionally, they noted that labral pathology on preoperative MRI had no impact on the clinical outcomes in the study. The PAO alone group demonstrated 55% of patients with preoperative Labral tear on MRI. Only 1 patient (1.1%) in the PAO alone group underwent labral repair. Thus, they argue that PAO alone, without hip arthroscopy, demonstrated similar outcomes without the time and risks of hip arthroscopy. They do acknowledge that longer follow-up (greater than the 1 year in their study) is needed to fully understand the difference between PAO alone compared to combined PAO and hip arthroscopy. Additionally, it was noted that in the PAO alone cohort, 35% of patients underwent an open CAM resection with 16% of total patients undergoing a subspine decompression.[26] This stands to question if the PAO still requires a CAM and/or subspine decompression to achieve maximal results in the way of PROMs. If so, one might argue that these procedures could be performed arthroscopically, which might use smaller capsulotomies than those required to perform these surgeries through an open approach. Longer follow-up and further evidence are needed to fully appreciate the difference in outcomes between groups.

SUMMARY

Combined hip arthroscopy and PAO is associated with improved outcomes in patient who have symptomatic hip dysplasia with concomitant intra-articular or extra-articular hip pathology. Modifications to the arthroscopic procedure include illiocapsularis dissection from the underlying capsule after capsular closure to aid in and begin the dissection for the PAO. When used in combination, these procedures have been shown to be safe and effective in addressing symptomatic dysplasia.

CLINICS CARE POINTS

- Consider combining PAO with concurrent hip arthroscopy due to the high rate of intraarticular pathology associated with hip dysplasia.
- Arthroscopic elevation of the iliocapsularis can be performed after capsular closure to aid in the PAO dissection.
- Combined hip arthroscopy and PAO has been associated with good clinical outcomes.

DISCLOSURE

B. Ronna, MD: None, A. Chrumka, MD- None. A. Stryker: Type: Other Professional Activities. International Hip Preservation Society: Type: Board of Directors or committee member Self. American Journal of Sports Medicine, Journal of Hip Preservation Surgery, Arthroscopy Journal, Video Journal of Sports Medicine: Type: Editorial or governing board Self.

SUPPLEMENTARY DATA

Supplementary data to this article can be found online at https://doi.org/10.1016/j.csm.2026.03.008.

REFERENCES

1. LaPrade MD, Melugin HP, Hale RF, et al. Incidence of hip dysplasia diagnosis in young patients with hip pain: a geographic population cohort analysis. Orthop J Sports Med 2021;9(3). https://doi.org/10.1177/2325967121989087.
2. Kyin C, Maldonado DR, Go CC, et al. Mid- to long-term outcomes of hip arthroscopy: a systematic review. Arthrosc J Arthrosc Relat Surg 2021;37(3):1011–25.
3. Zusmanovich M, Haselman W, Serrano B, et al. The incidence of hip arthroscopy in patients with femoroacetabular impingement syndrome and labral pathology increased by 85% between 2011 and 2018 in the United States. Arthrosc J Arthrosc Relat Surg 2022;38(1):82–7.
4. Murata Y, Uchida S, Utsunomiya H, et al. A comparison of clinical outcome between athletes and nonathletes undergoing hip arthroscopy for femoroacetabular impingement. Clin J Sport Med 2017;27(4):349–56.

5. Wilson ES, Wagner KR, Spiker AM. Borderline hip dysplasia - best treated with hip arthroscopy or periacetabular osteotomy? Curr Rev Musculoskelet Med 2024;17(12):538–47.
6. Clohisy JC, Dobson MA, Robison JF, et al. Radiographic structural abnormalities associated with premature, natural hip-joint failure. J Bone Joint Surg 2011;93-(Supplement_2):3–9.
7. Rankin AT, Bleakley CM, Cullen M. Hip joint pathology as a leading cause of groin pain in the sporting population. Am J Sports Med 2015;43(7):1698–703.
8. Gala L, Clohisy JC, Beaulé PE. Hip dysplasia in the young adult. J Bone Joint Surg 2016;98(1):63–73.
9. Wilkin GP, Ibrahim MM, Smit KM, et al. A contemporary definition of hip dysplasia and structural instability: toward a comprehensive classification for acetabular dysplasia. J Arthroplast 2017;32(9):S20–7.
10. Clohisy JC, Carlisle JC, Beaulé PE, et al. A systematic approach to the plain radiographic evaluation of the young adult hip. J Bone Joint Surg 2008;90-(Supplement_4):47–66.
11. Smith JT, Jee Y, Daley E, et al. Can the femoro-epiphyseal acetabular roof (FEAR) index be used to Distinguish dysplasia from impingement? Clin Orthop Relat Res 2021;479(5):962–71.
12. Ganz R, Klaue K, Vinh TS, et al. A new periacetabular osteotomy for the treatment of hip dysplasias. Technique and preliminary results. Clin Orthop Relat Res 1988; 232:26–36.
13. Büchler L, Beck M. Periacetabular osteotomy: a review of Swiss experience. Curr Rev Musculoskelet Med 2014;7(4):330–6.
14. Wells J, Schoenecker P, Duncan S, et al. Intermediate-term hip survivorship and patient-reported outcomes of periacetabular osteotomy. J Bone Joint Surg 2018; 100(3):218–25.
15. Zaltz I, Baca G, Kim YJ, et al. Complications associated with the periacetabular osteotomy. J Bone Joint Surg 2014;96(23):1967–74.
16. Clohisy JC, Ackerman J, Baca G, et al. Patient-reported outcomes of periacetabular osteotomy from the prospective ANCHOR cohort study. J Bone Joint Surg 2017;99(1):33–41.
17. van Bergayk AB, Garbuz DS. Quality of life and sports-specific outcomes after Bernese periacetabular osteotomy. J Bone Joint Surg 2002;84(3):339–43.
18. Nepple JJ, Carlisle JC, Nunley RM, et al. Clinical and radiographic predictors of intra-articular hip disease in arthroscopy. Am J Sports Med 2011;39(2):296–303.
19. Dorrell J, Catterall A. The torn acetabular labrum. J Bone Joint Surg Br 1986;68-B-(3):400–3.
20. Domb BG, Lareau JM, Baydoun H, et al. Is intraarticular pathology common in patients with hip dysplasia undergoing periacetabular osteotomy? Clin Orthop Relat Res 2014;472(2):674–80.
21. Redmond JM, Gupta A, Stake CE, et al. The prevalence of hip labral and chondral lesions identified by method of detection during periacetabular osteotomy: arthroscopy versus arthrotomy. Arthrosc J Arthrosc Relat Surg 2014;30(3):382–8.
22. Kohno Y, Nakashima Y, Hatano T, et al. High prevalence of cam deformity in dysplastic hips: a three-dimensional CT study. J Orthop Res 2016;34(9):1613–9.
23. Domb B, LaReau J, Redmond JM, et al. Combined hip arthroscopy and periacetabular osteotomy: indications, advantages, technique, and complications. Arthrosc Tech 2014;3(1):e95–100.
24. Ricciardi BF, Mayer SW, Fields KG, et al. Patient characteristics and early functional outcomes of combined arthroscopic labral refixation and periacetabular

osteotomy for symptomatic acetabular dysplasia. Am J Sports Med 2016;44(10): 2518–25.
25. Nakayama H, Fukunishi S, Fukui T, et al. Arthroscopic labral repair concomitantly performed with curved periacetabular osteotomy. Knee Surg Sports Traumatol Arthrosc 2014;22(4):938–41.
26. Beaulé PE, Verhaegen JCF, Clohisy JC, et al. The otto aufranc award: does hip arthroscopy at the time of periacetabular osteotomy improve the clinical outcome for the treatment of hip dysplasia? A multicenter randomized clinical trial. J Arthroplast 2024;39(9):S9–16.
27. Verhaegen J, Salih S, Thiagarajah S, et al. Is a periacetabular osteotomy as efficacious in retroversion as it is in dysplasia? : the role of femoral anteversion on outcome. Bone Jt Open 2021;2(9):757–64.
28. Fujii M, Nakashima Y, Jingushi S, et al. Intraarticular findings in symptomatic developmental dysplasia of the hip. J Pediatr Orthop 2009;29(1):9–13.
29. Frank JM, Harris JD, Erickson BJ, et al. Prevalence of femoroacetabular impingement imaging findings in asymptomatic volunteers: a systematic review. Arthrosc J Arthrosc Relat Surg 2015;31(6):1199–204.
30. Maldonado DR, LaReau JM, Perets I, et al. Outcomes of hip arthroscopy with concomitant periacetabular osteotomy, minimum 5-Year Follow-Up. Arthrosc J Arthrosc Relat Surg 2019;35(3):826–34.
31. Jimenez AE, Lee MS, Owens JS, et al. Athletes undergoing concomitant hip arthroscopy and periacetabular osteotomy demonstrate greater than 80% return-to-sport rate at 2-Year minimum Follow-Up. Arthrosc J Arthrosc Relat Surg 2022;38(9):2649–58.
32. Novais EN, Ferraro SL, Miller P, et al. Periacetabular osteotomy for symptomatic acetabular dysplasia in patients ≥40 years old. J Bone Joint Surg 2023;105(15): 1175–81.
33. Anderson LA, Wylie JD, Kapron C, et al. The incidence of subsequent hip arthroscopy after rectus-sparing periacetabular osteotomy. Bone Joint J 2024;106-B(5 Supple B):17–24.
34. Laboudie P, Dymond T, Kreviazuk C, et al. Hip arthroscopy after periacetabular osteotomy for acetabular dysplasia – incidence and clinical outcome. BMC Musculoskelet Disord 2022;23(1):659.
35. Spiker AM, Turner EHG, Gans I, et al. Combined hip arthroscopy and periacetabular osteotomy (PAO): technical focus on arthroscopically elevating the iliocapsularis and performing the open PAO. Arthrosc Tech 2021;10(10):e2293–302.
36. Spiker AM, Gumersell KR, Sink EL, et al. Modifications to the hip arthroscopy technique when performing combined hip arthroscopy and periacetabular osteotomy. Arthrosc Tech 2017;6(5):e1857–63.
37. Sabbag CM, Nepple JJ, Pascual-Garrido C, et al. The addition of hip arthroscopy to periacetabular osteotomy does not increase complication rates: a prospective case series. Am J Sports Med 2019;47(3):543–51.

Arthroscopic Hip Capsular Reconstruction

John J. Kelly, MD, Aaron J. Krych, MD, Mario Hevesi, MD, PhD*

KEYWORDS

• Hip capsular reconstruction • Microinstability • Hip capsulotomy • Hip preservation • Dermal allograft • Iliotibial bad graft • Achilles allograft

KEY POINTS

- Hip microinstability is an increasingly recognized source of hip pain and dysfunction, often resulting from capsular insufficiency after hip arthroscopy or in the setting of generalized ligamentous laxity.
- The iliofemoral ligament is the most critical static stabilizer of the hip; its compromise during capsulotomy can significantly reduce distractive resistance and predispose to instability.
- Early identification and management of microinstability—preferably through capsular preservation and repair at the time of the index procedure—remain essential to preventing long-term morbidity.
- Capsular reconstruction, using grafts such as iliotibial band, dermal allograft, or Achilles tendon, can restore hip stability in cases of irreparable capsular deficiency.
- Evidence supports improved patient-reported outcomes with capsular closure or reconstruction, but long-term comparative data and refined surgical indications are still needed for the latter.

Video content accompanies this article at http://www.sportsmed.theclinics.com.

INTRODUCTION

Hip microinstability is increasingly recognized as a distinct pathologic entity and a potential source of chronic pain and dysfunction.[1] Historically, the hip was considered inherently stable due to its deep, congruent bony architecture and the compressive forces generated by surrounding musculature. However, mounting evidence demonstrates that unrecognized microinstability can overload intra-articular structures—particularly the labrum and articular cartilage—leading to labral hypertrophy, chondral injury, and progressive degeneration.[2–4]

Department of Orthopedic Surgery and Sports Medicine, Mayo Clinic, 200 First St SW, Rochester, MN, USA
* Corresponding author.
E-mail address: hevesi.mario@mayo.edu

Clin Sports Med 45 (2026) 675–691
https://doi.org/10.1016/j.csm.2026.01.003 sportsmed.theclinics.com

Abbreviations	
IFL	Iliofemoral ligament
PROM	patient-reported outcomes measure
ROM	ranges of motion

Risk factors for hip instability include acetabular dysplasia, abnormal femoral and/or acetabular version, loss of the suction seal due to labral damage, generalized ligamentous laxity (eg, Ehlers–Danlos syndrome or other connective tissue disorders), and sports requiring extreme ranges of motion (ROM) and torsional loading, such as gymnastics, ballet, and golf.[5–7] Furthermore, and of specific interest to this article, iatrogenic capsular insufficiency following arthroscopy has become an increasingly recognized contributor of instability.[8]

Over the past 2 decades, the incidence of both periacetabular osteotomy and hip arthroscopy has risen, reflecting a growing emphasis on joint preservation in patients with dysplasia, femoroacetabular impingement, and other hip pathologies.[9] This shift has fueled interest in capsuloligamentous contributions to stability—particularly as arthroscopic techniques necessarily involve capsular violation.[10,11] The recognition of iatrogenic instability has driven significant research into optimal capsular management, culminating in advanced techniques such as capsular reconstruction for cases in which native tissue is insufficient.[8,12,13] However, ultimately, prevention of microinstability through meticulous capsular preservation and repair at the index procedure remains paramount.

This article aims to review current concepts in hip capsular reconstruction in the setting of microinstability, including relevant anatomy, the etiologies and diagnosis of microinstability, surgical indications, reconstructive techniques, and future directions. While growing biomechanical and early clinical evidence supports capsular reconstruction in selected cases, there is limited literature supporting optimal indications, techniques, and long-term outcomes.

RELEVANT ANATOMY

Hip stability is maintained through a combination of osseous architecture, static soft tissue restraints, and dynamic muscular support. The bony configuration—comprising the spherical femoral head and concentric acetabulum—provides inherent stability, particularly when acetabular coverage and version are appropriate.[1,2,14]

Static stabilizers include the labrum, the joint capsule, and 3 primary capsular ligaments:

- Iliofemoral ligament (IFL): Y-shaped, originating just inferior to the anterior inferior iliac spine and inserting along the femoral intertrochanteric line. It is the strongest ligament of the hip and the most frequently implicated in microinstability. The IFL resists extension, external rotation, and internal rotation in extension. During arthroscopy, it is transected perpendicularly during an interportal capsulotomy and both longitudinally and perpendicularly during a T-capsulotomy.[15]
- Pubofemoral ligament: Originates from the pubis and blends with the medial IFL before inserting along the femoral intertrochanteric line. It limits external rotation and abduction.[15]
- Ischiofemoral ligament: Blends with the posterior capsule, connecting the posterior acetabulum to the posterior femoral neck. It restricts internal rotation in both flexion and extension.[15]

The zona orbicularis is a circumferential thickening of the capsule that encircles the femoral neck and resists distraction.[16]

The ligamentum teres is less commonly considered a primary stabilizer but may play a more important role in dysplastic hips lacking adequate acetabular coverage. It resists external rotation in flexion and internal rotation in extension and contains free nerve endings, making it a potential pain generator when torn. While its role in microinstability remains controversial, traumatic injury to the ligamentum teres—such as during hip dislocation—has been associated with subsequent instability symptoms in a subset of patients.[16,17]

Dynamic stabilizers—including the deep external rotators, gluteus medius, and gluteus minimus—contribute to joint stability by providing compressive forces across the joint.[6]

MICROINSTABILITY

Etiology and Pathogenesis

A thorough understanding of the underlying etiology of hip microinstability is fundamental to selecting the most appropriate management strategy. Although microinstability may arise from a variety of etiologies, patients most suitable for capsular reconstruction often present with capsular insufficiency secondary to a prior hip procedure involving capsulotomy or a documented history of connective tissue disorder.[18]

Iatrogenic capsular insufficiency

Hip arthroscopy necessitates joint distraction to access intra-articular pathology. To facilitate adequate visualization and create a working environment, many surgeons perform an interportal capsulotomy extending from the mid-anterior to the anterolateral portal, transecting the IFL perpendicularly. Others prefer a T-shaped capsulotomy, incorporating a longitudinal limb through the IFL to achieve greater exposure. Although these techniques enhance access, they compromise the capsule's intrinsic stabilizing function.[11,19]

Extended capsulotomy without subsequent repair has been associated with postoperative instability and, in some cases, frank dislocation, with reported 1 year dislocation rates of approximately 0.6%.[20] Postoperative subluxation or dislocation often occurs in the presence of concomitant pathology, including labral insufficiency, acetabular undercoverage, and iliopsoas tenotomy, and most commonly presents anteriorly with hip extension and external rotation. Patients at increased risk include females, those with acetabular dysplasia, and individuals with conditions predisposing to generalized ligamentous laxity.[21]

Of note, even patients without frank instability likely experience sequelae of incomplete capsular closure. In Frank and colleagues' 2014 study, patients undergoing partial repair of a T-capsulotomy experienced statistically inferior subjective outcomes at 6, 12, and 30 month postoperatively as well as increased revision arthroscopy rates (13% vs 0%) as compared to patients undergoing complete repair.[22]

Other contributing factors

In addition to iatrogenic causes, microinstability may occur in patients with:

- Generalized ligamentous laxity (eg, Ehler's Danlos Syndrome or connective tissue disorders)
- Repetitive microtrauma from sports requiring extreme motion and torsional loading
- Traumatic capsular injury not amenable to primary repair

In these cases, the loss of capsular tension and continuity disrupts the hip's ability to resist distraction, rotation, and translation, leading to symptoms and functional decline.[21,23]

Abnormal femoral version is another important and well-recognized factor contributing to hip instability and microinstability. Excessive femoral anteversion positions the femoral head in relative internal rotation, thereby increasing reliance on the anterior capsule and, in particular, the IFL for restraint.[4] This heightened mechanical demand may result in progressive stretching or attenuation of the anterior capsule, which can manifest clinically as microinstability. Moreover, increased anteversion has been correlated with decreased anterior capsular thickness, further predisposing affected patients to symptomatic anterior instability.[24]

RECONSTRUCTION

Recognition of these risks has driven the adoption of routine capsular closure, which is associated with improved patient reported outcomes measures (PROMs) and lower reoperation rates. Closure also allows surgeons to perform capsular plication when laxity or redundancy is identified intraoperatively. However, in revision cases or after excessive tissue resection, primary repair may not be possible—making capsular reconstruction necessary to restore stability.[8,11,25]

Patient Assessment

Evaluating a patient for possible capsular reconstruction in the setting of hip microinstability requires a systematic approach that integrates history, physical examination, and imaging. Because symptoms can be subtle and nonspecific, maintaining a high index of suspicion is critical—especially in patients with known risk factors.

History

Patients often present with progressive, deep-seated groin or hip pain, sometimes accompanied by mechanical symptoms such as popping or locking. A subset may describe a subjective sense of instability or apprehension during activities that place the hip in extension, external rotation, or extreme abduction.

Microinstability should be suspected in:

- Female patients
- Individuals with prior hip arthroscopy
- Athletes in sports requiring excessive torsional loading (eg, ballet, golf, gymnastics)
- Patients with known ligamentous laxity or connective tissue disorders

Physical Examination

Generalized ligamentous laxity can be assessed using the Beighton score. Preoperative documentation of baseline hip ROM is important, as increased rotation or extension may indicate capsular laxity.[26]

Several provocative maneuvers can aid in confirming the diagnosis of hip microinstability. The three most widely accepted are as follows:

1. Prone External Rotation Test—Highest specificity (~98%) for microinstability.
2. Abduction–Extension–External Rotation (AB–ER) Test—Reproduces instability symptoms in extension and abduction.
3. Anterior Apprehension Test—Elicits discomfort or apprehension with the hip in extension and external rotation.

4. Bounce test—External rotation with release results in less “spring” back, indicating loss of anterior capsular restraint (Video 1).

A positive result on all 3 tests confers approximately a 95% likelihood of confirming microinstability intraoperatively.[27]

Imaging

Radiographs

Plain radiographs are the first step in evaluating suspected microinstability, both to identify capsuloligamentous pathology and to rule out bony abnormalities that would not benefit from capsular reconstruction alone.

Standard views include:

- Supine AP pelvis—Evaluate lateral center-edge angle (dysplasia defined as <20°–25°) and acetabular retroversion (posterior wall sign, ischial spine sign) and measure the Tönnis angle (>10° suggests dysplasia).
- Lateral Dunn view—Assess femoral head–neck morphology.
- False profile view—Evaluate anterior coverage with anterior center-edge angle (<20° suggests dysplasia)

Additional radiographic indicators of instability include the *cliff sign* and the *femoral epiphyseal acetabular roof* index.[28–30] Fluoroscopic arthrogram can also provide valuable diagnostic information by demonstrating fluid extravasation beyond the joint confines (**Fig. 1**A, B).

MRI/MR arthrogram

Magnetic resonance arthrography is particularly valuable in detecting capsular defects, redundancy, and associated soft tissue abnormalities (**Fig. 2**A–E).

Key findings include as follows:

- Anterior hip joint recess sign—An area lateral to the zona orbicularis measuring greater than 5 mm on axial imaging suggests microinstability and is often accompanied by capsular thinning (<3 mm).[31]
- Posteroinferior crescent sign—A crescent-shaped accumulation of contrast in the posteroinferior joint space on ≥2 imaging planes, consistent with capsular laxity or detachment.[32]

These imaging findings, when integrated with a thorough clinical examination, are critical in determining the appropriateness of surgical versus nonsurgical management strategies.

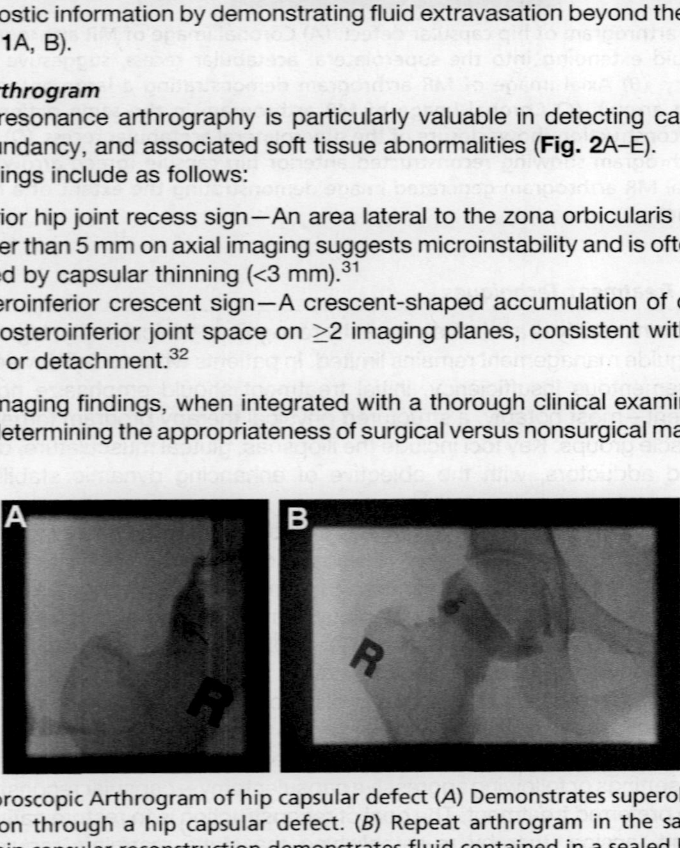

Fig. 1. Fluoroscopic Arthrogram of hip capsular defect (*A*) Demonstrates superolateral fluid extravasation through a hip capsular defect. (*B*) Repeat arthrogram in the same patient following hip capsular reconstruction demonstrates fluid contained in a sealed hip capsule.

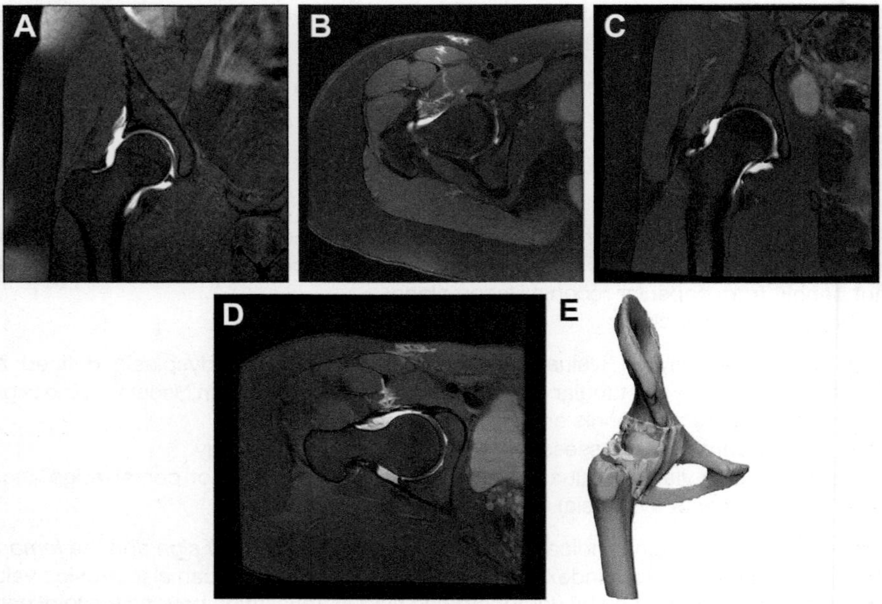

Fig. 2. MR arthrogram of hip capsular defect: (*A*) Coronal image of MR arthrogram demonstrating fluid extending into the superolateral acetabular recess, suggestive of capsular insufficiency. (*B*) Axial image of MR arthrogram demonstrating a large anterior capsular defect (*red arrow*). (*C*) Coronal image of MR arthrogram in the same patient following capsular reconstruction shows closure of the superolateral acetabular recess. (*D*) Axial image of MRI arthrogram showing reconstructed anterior hip capsule (*green arrow*). (*E*) Three-dimensional MR arthrogram generated image demonstrating the extent of a hip capsular defect (*blue*).

Emerging Treatment Techniques

As hip microinstability is a relatively recently recognized clinical entity, high-quality evidence to guide management remains limited. In patients without definitive evidence of capsuloligamentous insufficiency, initial treatment should emphasize nonoperative management—most notably, a structured physical therapy program targeting periarticular muscle groups. Key foci include the iliopsoas, gluteal musculature, deep hip rotators, and adductors, with the objective of enhancing dynamic stability through improved neuromuscular control.[33]

Patients who fail to achieve symptomatic improvement with conservative measures, or those demonstrating clear objective signs of capsular deficiency on imaging, may be considered for surgical intervention. In primary cases, operative management should first address concomitant pathology that may contribute to instability, such as labral tears or osseous abnormalities. Capsular closure is essential in these situations, and when capsular redundancy or laxity is present—particularly in patients with generalized ligamentous laxity—capsular plication or thermal capsulorrhaphy may be warranted.[1,6,8]

In cases where the capsule is deficient or irreparable—most commonly encountered in revision settings or following aggressive capsulectomy—capsular reconstruction becomes the preferred treatment. The goal of reconstruction is to restore native capsular volume and tension, thereby re-establishing the static restraints required for hip stability. Both open and arthroscopic techniques have been described, although comparative outcome data between these approaches are currently lacking.[12,14]

Arthroscopic capsular reconstruction offers advantages over open techniques, including the ability to address intra-articular pathology with less soft tissue disruption, reduced morbidity, and faster recovery.[11,25] The arthroscopic approach allows precise anchor placement and graft fixation under direct visualization and is generally favored in revision cases, with open reconstruction reserved for severe deficiency or complex scenarios.[34] While comparative data remain limited, current evidence and practice trends support arthroscopy as the preferred approach.

Intraoperative Considerations

During surgery for suspected hip microinstability—particularly in the revision setting—several key intraoperative assessments can aid in confirming the diagnosis and guiding management. These assessments include examination under anesthesia,[35] ease of distraction,[6] chondrolabral pathology patterns,[36] and ligamentum teres integrity[37] are listed in further detail in **Table 1**.

HIP CAPSULAR RECONSTRUCTION

Graft Selection

Multiple graft options have been described for hip capsular reconstruction, each with distinct biomechanical properties, handling characteristics, and levels of supporting evidence. Selection is influenced by surgeon preference, graft availability, patient-specific factors, and intraoperative findings. **Table 2** summarizes commonly used graft types, key literature, and reported outcomes or technical considerations to provide a comparative framework for decision-making.

Technical Variations

Several techniques have been described to optimize graft delivery,[43,44] fixation, and coverage in hip capsular reconstruction.[45–54]

Authors' preferred technique

The patient is positioned supine on a hip distraction table with traction applied under fluoroscopic guidance (see Video 1).[46] After establishing anterolateral and modified

Table 1
Intraoperative considerations in suspected hip microinstability

Assessment	Purpose/Findings	Key Notes
Examination Under Anesthesia (EUA)	Compare ROM in with the preoperative baseline or contralateral limb	Excessive rotation or extension may indicate capsular insufficiency
Ease of Distraction	Fluoroscopic assessment of joint distractibility	Increased ease of distractibility suggests laxity
Chondrolabral Pathology Patterns	Identify mechanisms of instability based on injury location	Isolated anterior or lateral injury → microinstability; anterolateral damage → often FAI-related
Ligamentum Teres Integrity	Assess for partial or complete tearing	Frequently encountered in patients with instability

Table 2
Graft selection and key literature in hip capsular reconstruction

Graft Type	Key References	Findings/Outcomes
Iliotibial Band (ITB) Allograft	Fagotti et al,[38] 2018—cadaveric	Improved distractive stability at time zero; limited by lack of biological healing assessment
	Fagotti et al,[39] 2019—clinical comparative	Short-term PROs favored ITB allograft over dermal allograft; survivorship similar
	Ruzbarsky et al,[25]—midterm	86% survivorship free of THA at 3 y; 10 revisions (6 conversions to THA at mean 2 y, 4 revision hip arthroscopy for capsulolabral adhesions)
ITB Autograft/ Achilles Tendon Allograft	Pasic et al,[40] 2020—cadaveric	ITB autograft had comparable rotational/translational stability to Achilles allograft; distraction not assessed
	Mei-Dan et al,[41] 2015—Achilles Allograft	Recommend using the midportion of tendon, folded to achieve consistent thickness; preop MRI to facilitate graft sizing
Dermal Allograft	Jacobsen et al,[42] 2020—cadaveric	Restored distractive resistance to within 5% of the native capsule
	Jimenez et al,[12] 2021—systematic review	Improved torsional and distractive stability approximating native mechanics

mid-anterior portals, the capsule is defined using a shaver and radiofrequency ablator, with adhesions lysed to re-establish native tissue planes (**Fig. 3**A–C). Any intra-articular work such as labral repair is performed first. Remaining under traction in full extension with 15° internal rotation, the acetabular rim is then prepared, and suture anchors are placed approximately 3 mm proximal to labral anchors, spaced every 10 to 15 mm across the capsular defect (**Fig. 4**). Sutures near the indirect head of the rectus femoris are passed in a horizontal mattress configuration

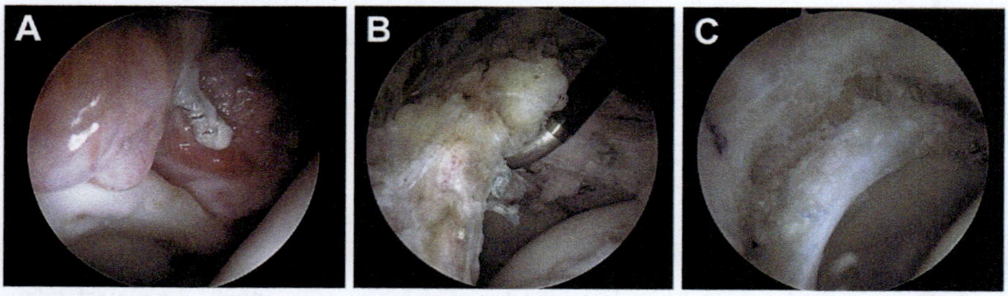

Fig. 3. Arthroscopic visualization of capsular defect and adhesions (*A*) viewing from an anterolateral portal in a right hip, one can appreciate a large anterior capsular defect. (*B*) View from anterolateral portal demonstrating significant labral adhesions that may be encountered in the revision setting. (*C*) View from anterolateral portal demonstrating hip joint and acetabular rim following appropriate lysis of adhesions.

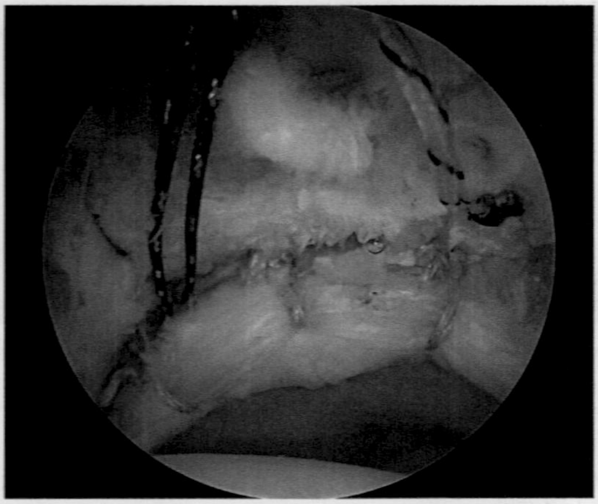

Fig. 4. Preparation for rectus overlay technique. Following labral repair or reconstruction, pre-loaded anchors are placed in the acetabular rim 10 to 15 mm apart, spanning the width of the capsule defect.

through the tendon in preparation for reconstruction reinforcement with rectus overlay (**Fig. 5**).

Traction is removed. The distal capsule is exposed, mobilized, and traction sutures are placed to control the leaflet. The capsular defect is measured, and a dermal allograft is cut 1 cm larger in each dimension (**Fig. 6**A, B). A horizontal mattress suture is placed in the distal cuff, and all proximal and distal sutures are retrieved through the distal anterolateral accessory portal, ensuring a tangle-free corridor. Sutures are sequentially passed through the graft on the back table, which is then shuttled and docked arthroscopically, tying down the medial, central, and lateral anchors, followed by the distal leaflet. The graft is further secured to the native capsule circumferentially

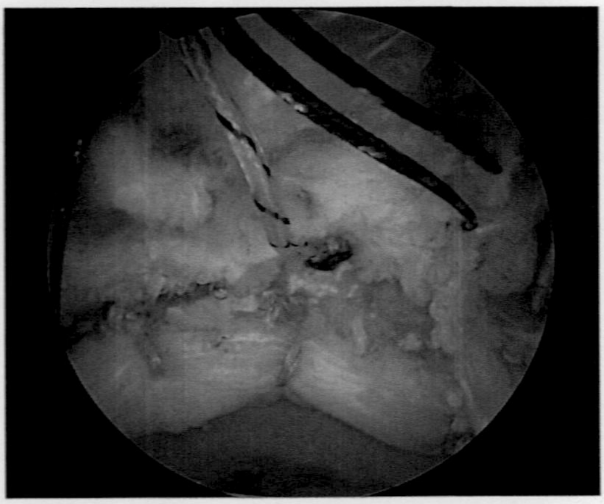

Fig. 5. Preparation for rectus overlay technique. Both limbs from one of two suture pairs in the medial suture anchor are placed in a horizontal mattress fashion through the indirect head of the rectus femoris (*black sutures*) and placed aside for later incorporation into the reconstructed hip capsule.

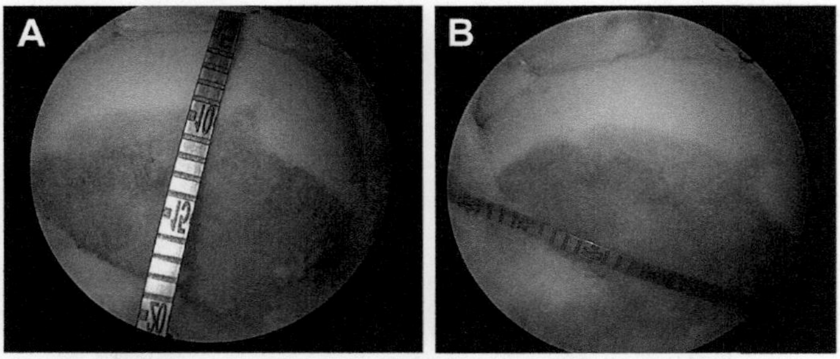

Fig. 6. Graft size measurement. The length (*A*) and width (*B*) of the defect are measured arthroscopically and a graft 1 cm larger in each direction is prepared to ensure adequate overlap with the native capsule.

(**Fig. 7**). The authors find that graft passage and fixation are best accomplished with the hip fully extended (0°) and in neutral rotation to allow for a tension-free repair.

Finally, the rectus overlay is completed by tying sutures previously passed through the rectus femoris tendon, bringing it down in a "pants-over-vest" manner to reinforce the reconstruction. Portals are closed in a layered fashion, and patients are placed in a hip brace with partial weightbearing (25%) and limited hip motion for 6 weeks, followed by structured physical therapy.

Postoperative Rehabilitation

To protect the integrity of the reconstruction, most technique guidelines recommend a period of partial weight-bearing and restricted ROM for 2 to 6 weeks postoperatively. Movements that place excessive stress on the anterior capsule—particularly external rotation, extension, and abduction—should be avoided during this phase. While physical therapy is typically initiated early to promote mobility and neuromuscular control, return to high-impact activities or sport is generally deferred until approximately 4 to 6 months following surgery.[25,43,46]

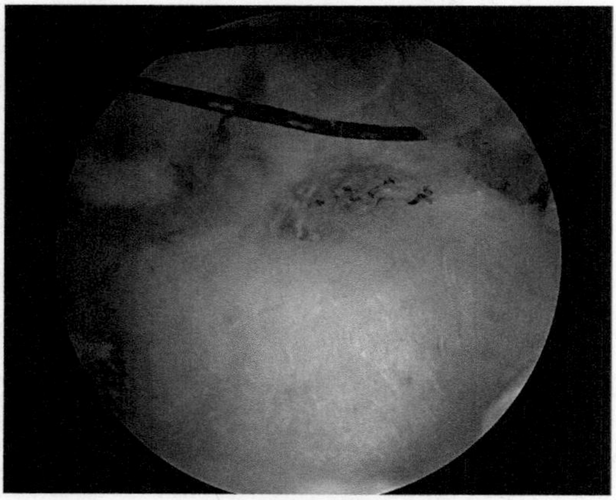

Fig. 7. Dermal allograft fixation. The dermal allograft is introduced intra-articularly, secured proximally to the acetabular rim anchors and distally to the native capsule, with additional medial and lateral fixation to achieve circumferential stability. The previously placed rectus tendon sutures are then tied down to the graft.

Table 3
Pearls and pitfalls to hip capsular reconstruction

	Pearls	Pitfalls
Graft Sizing	Oversizing graft (approximately 1 cm in length and width) to ensure overlap with the remaining native capsule distally Consider preoperative templating defect size on MRI and confirm with intraoperative measurement	Undersized grafts may result in over-tensioning resulting in restricting ROM, pain or early failure. Additionally, incomplete defect coverage may result in residual instability
Tissue Preparation	Perform thorough lysis of adhesions to reestablish native tissue planes and fully expose capsular defect	Failure to develop enough acetabular rim proximally may lead to having to work around labral repair, exposing it to injury
Operative Sequence	Address labral pathology prior to placing acetabular rim anchors for capsular reconstruction	Failure to plan out anchor locations for both labral repair and capsular reconstruction may lead to loss of real estate, obstructing anchor placement for capsular fixation
Graft Passage	Develop a technique for consistent, appropriate graft passage to ensure the graft is delivered easily and in the appropriate plane	Graft flipping or entanglement with sutures may lead to prolonged operative times
Suture Management	Maintain clear suture organization and consider the use of accessory portals to avoid soft tissue bridges or suture tangles	Interposed tissue may prevent direct apposition of the graft to the native capsule, leading to persistent defects or instability

DISCUSSION

Successful hip capsular reconstruction requires meticulous attention to technical detail, as small errors in graft sizing, fixation sequence, or suture management can compromise stability and clinical outcomes. Several operative strategies have been proposed to optimize graft integration, restore capsular tension, and minimize complications. **Table 3** outlines key pearls and common pitfalls to serve as a quick intraoperative reference.

Hip capsular reconstruction offers the potential to restore stability in cases of irreparable capsular deficiency; however, prevention of microinstability—through meticulous capsular preservation and repair at the index procedure—remains the most critical determinant of long-term hip function. The IFL, particularly its lateral arm, serves as the primary restraint to external rotation in flexion and anterior translation, with both arms contributing to resistance against internal rotation in neutral and extension.[15,17,28]

Biomechanical evidence demonstrates that enlargement of an interportal capsulotomy significantly reduces axial distractive resistance, whereas the addition of a longitudinal T-limb to an already large interportal incision yields minimal further loss.[19]

Complete capsular repair restores native distractive resistance and normalizes hip kinematics, while incomplete or failed repair leaves the joint vulnerable to recurrent microinstability.[55]

Technical reviews emphasize tailoring capsular management to the specific pathology. In cases of subspine impingement—although relatively uncommon—careful consideration is necessary when performing superior acetabular rim preparation and labral repair, as these maneuvers may necessitate anterior capsular elevation. However, unless subspine decompression is indicated, extensive capsular elevation near the 2:00 to 3:00 position may be able to be avoided to preserve the capsulolabral junction and minimize disruption of the IFL.[11,56]

Knowledge of the anatomic relationship between the IFL and the acetabular clock face (approximately 12:30–3:00) is critical in guiding portal placement to protect ligament integrity.[57,58] When increased exposure is essential, extending a longitudinal capsulotomy, forming a T-capsulotomy, may better maintain ligamentous continuity than extending the interportal, which runs perpendicular to the ligament.[59]

Additionally, the use of a periportal capsulotomy has been described as a technique to preserve more of the IFL. Two-year clinical outcome data from this cohort demonstrated no cases of postoperative instability requiring capsular reconstruction, irrespective of whether the periportal capsulotomy sites were repaired.[60] Although biomechanical studies revealed a slight increase in hip distraction distance when periportal capsulotomies were left unrepaired, this difference was minimal.[48,61]

Future Directions

Although early outcomes of hip capsular reconstruction are encouraging, the procedure remains in its relative infancy, and several key questions warrant further investigation:

- Comparative Effectiveness: Well-designed, adequately powered, long-term comparative studies are needed to evaluate iliotibial band, dermal allograft, and Achilles tendon grafts head-to-head, with follow-up extending beyond 5 to 10 years.
- Cost and Survivorship: Research should address not only clinical efficacy but also cost-effectiveness, reoperation rates, and long-term survivorship.
- Indication Refinement: Advances in the phenotyping of hip microinstability and clearer criteria for "reconstructability" will improve patient selection and enhance reproducibility.
- Outcomes should extend beyond PROMS to include return-to-sport and return-to-work rates, graft incorporation and remodeling data, and comprehensive complication profiles.
- Biomechanical Insights: Further biomechanical studies are necessary to refine graft tensioning protocols, fixation techniques, and biologic augmentation strategies to optimize integration and long-term durability.

SUMMARY

Hip microinstability, once underappreciated, is now recognized as a significant contributor to hip pain and dysfunction, especially after arthroscopic capsulotomy. The IFL plays a pivotal role in stability, and its preservation is critical. When repair is not possible, capsular reconstruction can restore joint mechanics, with promising early clinical results across several graft types. Rehabilitation protocols must protect the reconstruction during early healing while restoring dynamic stability. Future research should focus on refining indications, optimizing graft selection, and evaluating long-term outcomes beyond patient-reported measures.

CLINICS CARE POINTS

- Always evaluate pre- and intraoperative hip ROM and ease of distraction to identify potential instability.
- Preserve as much of the IFL as possible during capsulotomy, particularly as it relates to interportal capsulotomy length, in order to primarily maintain native stability.
- In revision cases or when native tissue is insufficient, consider capsular reconstruction to restore capsular tension and volume.
- Oversize the graft by ~1 cm in both dimensions to ensure adequate overlap with the native capsule and a secure seal.
- Complete labral repair before placing acetabular anchors for capsular reconstruction to avoid obstructing anchor placement.
- Limit hip extension and external rotation for the first 4 to 6 weeks postoperatively to protect the reconstruction.

DISCLOSURES

M. Hevesi reports a consulting or advisory relationship with DJO-Enovis, Arthrex, Moximed, Stryker, and Vericel and acknowledges editorial board privileges with the Journal of Cartilage and Joint Preservation. A.J. Krych reports a consulting or advisory relationship with Arthrex, board membership with Arthroscopy Association of North America and International Cartilage Repair Society and acknowledges editorial board privileges for Springer and American Journal of Sports Medicine.

SUPPLEMENTARY DATA

Supplementary data to this article can be found online at https://doi.org/10.1016/j.csm.2026.01.003.

REFERENCES

1. Safran MR. Microinstability of the hip-gaining acceptance. J Am Acad Orthop Surg 2019;27(1):12–22.
2. Dangin A, Tardy N, Wettstein M, et al. Microinstability of the hip: a review. Orthop Traumatol Surg Res OTSR 2016;102(8S):S301–9.
3. Han S, Alexander JW, Thomas VS, et al. Does capsular laxity lead to microinstability of the native hip? Am J Sports Med 2018;46(6):1315–23.
4. Johannsen AM, Behn AW, Shibata K, et al. The role of anterior capsular laxity in hip microinstability: a novel biomechanical model. Am J Sports Med 2019;47(5):1151–8.
5. Dumont GD. Hip instability: current concepts and treatment options. Clin Sports Med 2016;35(3):435–47.
6. Curtis DM, Murray IR, Money AJ, et al. Hip microinstability: understanding a newly defined hip pathology in young athletes. Arthrosc J Arthrosc Relat Surg 2022;38(2):211–3.
7. Hoffer AJ, Beel W, Ng KCG, et al. The contribution of soft tissue and bony stabilizers to the hip suction seal: a systematic review of biomechanical studies. Am J Sports Med 2024;52(10):2657–66.
8. Ortiz-Declet V, Mu B, Chen AW, et al. Should the capsule be repaired or plicated after hip arthroscopy for labral tears associated with femoroacetabular impingement

or instability? A systematic review. Arthrosc J Arthrosc Relat Surg 2018;34(1): 303–18.
9. Edelstein AI, Nepple JJ, Abu-Amer W, et al. What mid-term patient-reported outcome measure scores, reoperations, and complications are associated with concurrent hip arthroscopy and periacetabular osteotomy to treat dysplasia with associated intraarticular abnormalities? Clin Orthop 2021;479(5):1068–77.
10. Owens JS, Jimenez AE, Shapira J, et al. Capsular repair may improve outcomes in patients undergoing hip arthroscopy for femoroacetabular impingement: a systematic review of comparative outcome studies. Arthrosc J Arthrosc Relat Surg 2021;37(9):2975–90.
11. Beck EC, Suppauksorn S, Nho SJ. The role of comprehensive capsular management in hip arthroscopy for the treatment of femoroacetabular impingement syndrome. Arthrosc J Arthrosc Relat Surg 2020;36(1):9–11.
12. Jimenez AE, Owens JS, Shapira J, et al. Hip capsular management in patients with femoroacetabular impingement or microinstability: a systematic review of biomechanical studies. Arthrosc J Arthrosc Relat Surg 2021;37(8):2642–54.
13. Looney AM, McCann JA, Connolly PT, et al. Routine capsular closure with hip arthroscopic surgery results in superior outcomes: a systematic review and meta-analysis. Am J Sports Med 2022;50(7):2007–22.
14. Parvaresh KC, Rasio J, Azua E, et al. Hip instability in the athlete: anatomy, etiology, and management. Clin Sports Med 2021;40(2):289–300.
15. Myers CA, Register BC, Lertwanich P, et al. Role of the acetabular labrum and the iliofemoral ligament in hip stability: an in vitro biplane fluoroscopy study. Am J Sports Med 2011;39(Suppl):85S–91S.
16. Flores DV, Foster RCB, Sampaio ML, et al. Hip capsulolabral complex: anatomy, disease, MRI features, and postoperative appearance. Radiogr Rev Publ Radiol Soc N Am Inc 2024;44(2):e230144. https://doi.org/10.1148/rg.230144.
17. van Arkel RJ, Amis AA, Cobb JP, et al. The capsular ligaments provide more hip rotational restraint than the acetabular labrum and the ligamentum teres : an experimental study. Bone Jt J 2015;97-B(4):484–91.
18. Yeung M, Memon M, Simunovic N, et al. Gross instability after hip arthroscopy: an analysis of case reports evaluating surgical and patient factors. Arthrosc J Arthrosc Relat Surg 2016;32(6):1196–204.e1.
19. Weber AE, Neal WH, Mayer EN, et al. Vertical extension of the T-Capsulotomy incision in hip arthroscopic surgery does not affect the force required for hip distraction: effect of capsulotomy size, type, and subsequent repair. Am J Sports Med 2018;46(13):3127–33.
20. Duplantier NL, McCulloch PC, Nho SJ, et al. Hip dislocation or subluxation after hip arthroscopy: a systematic review. Arthrosc J Arthrosc Relat Surg 2016;32(7): 1428–34.
21. Metz AK, Featherall J, Froerer DL, et al. Female patients and decreased hip capsular thickness on magnetic resonance imaging associated with increased axial distraction distance on examination under anesthesia: an in vivo study. Arthrosc J Arthrosc Relat Surg 2022;38(12):3133–40.
22. Frank RM, Lee S, Bush-Joseph CA, et al. Improved outcomes after hip arthroscopic surgery in patients undergoing T-capsulotomy with complete repair versus partial repair for femoroacetabular impingement: a comparative matched-pair analysis. Am J Sports Med 2014;42(11):2634–42.
23. Kraeutler MJ, Terle PM, Malempati M, et al. Risk factors for failure of hip arthroscopy in patients with borderline dysplasia include a tönnis angle $\geq 15°$, age ≥ 40 to 42 years, female sex, anterior wall index <0.35, labral debridement, and

preexisting hip osteoarthritis: a systematic review. Arthrosc J Arthrosc Relat Surg 2025;41(7):2636–45.
24. Yang F, Shi Y, Zhang X, et al. Femoral anteversion is associated with a thinner anterior capsule in patients with femoroacetabular impingement syndrome. Arthrosc J Arthrosc Relat Surg 2024;40(1):71–7.
25. Ruzbarsky JJ, Seiter MN, Comfort SM, et al. Arthroscopic hip capsular reconstruction using iliotibial band allograft as a salvage option for unrepairable capsular defects demonstrates good survivorship and improved patient-reported outcomes. Arthrosc J Arthrosc Relat Surg 2022;38(7):2219–26.
26. Khanduja V, Darby N, O'Donnell J, et al, International Microinstability Expert Panel. Diagnosing hip microinstability: an international consensus study using the Delphi methodology. Knee Surg Sports Traumatol Arthrosc Off J ESSKA 2023;31(1):40–9.
27. Kalisvaart MM, Safran MR. Microinstability of the hip-it does exist: etiology, diagnosis and treatment. J Hip Preserv Surg 2015;2(2):123–35.
28. Wyatt M, Weidner J, Pfluger D, et al. The femoro-epiphyseal acetabular roof (FEAR) index: a new measurement associated with instability in borderline hip dysplasia? Clin Orthop 2017;475(3):861–9.
29. Guimarães JB, Arruda PHC, Cerezal L, et al. Hip microinstability: new concepts and comprehensive imaging evaluation. Radiogr Rev Publ Radiol Soc N Am Inc 2025;45(7):e240134. https://doi.org/10.1148/rg.240134.
30. Truntzer JN, Hoppe DJ, Shapiro LM, et al. Can the FEAR index be used to predict microinstability in patients undergoing hip arthroscopic surgery? Am J Sports Med 2019;47(13):3158–65.
31. Magerkurth O, Jacobson JA, Morag Y, et al. Capsular laxity of the hip: findings at magnetic resonance arthrography. Arthrosc J Arthrosc Relat Surg 2013;29(10):1615–22.
32. MacDonald AA, Blankenbaker DG, Brick MJ, et al. The posterior crescent sign on MRI and MR arthrography: is it a marker of hip dysplasia and instability? Skelet Radiol 2023;52(6):1127–35.
33. Ejnisman L, Elisman K, Safran MR. Effectiveness of nonoperative management of hip microinstability. Am J Sports Med 2022;50(4):1013–9.
34. Tahoun MF, Lizano-Díez X, Soler BC, et al. Superior outcomes after arthroscopic treatment of femoroacetabular impingement and labral tears with closed versus open capsule. Knee Surg Sports Traumatol Arthrosc Off J ESSKA 2023;31(10):4501–9.
35. Cohen D, Jean PO, Patel M, et al. Hip microinstability diagnosis and management: a systematic review. Knee Surg Sports Traumatol Arthrosc Off J ESSKA 2023;31(1):16–32.
36. Shibata KR, Matsuda S, Safran MR. Is there a distinct pattern to the acetabular labrum and articular cartilage damage in the non-dysplastic hip with instability? Knee Surg Sports Traumatol Arthrosc Off J ESSKA 2017;25(1):84–93.
37. Wu JY, Li W, Xu LY, et al. Ligamentum teres tears and increased combined anteversion are associated with hip microinstability in patients with borderline dysplasia. Arthrosc J Arthrosc Relat Surg 2024;40(3):745–51.
38. Fagotti L, Kemler BR, Utsunomiya H, et al. Effects of capsular reconstruction with an iliotibial band allograft on distractive stability of the hip joint: a biomechanical study. Am J Sports Med 2018;46(14):3429–36.
39. Fagotti L, Soares E, Bolia IK, et al. Early outcomes after arthroscopic hip capsular reconstruction using iliotibial band allograft versus dermal allograft. Arthrosc J Arthrosc Relat Surg 2019;35(3):778–86.

40. Pasic N, Burkhart TA, Baha P, et al. A biomechanical comparison of 2 hip capsular reconstruction techniques: iliotibial band autograft versus achilles tendon allograft. Am J Sports Med 2020;48(13):3288–95.
41. Mei-Dan O, Garabekyan T, McConkey M, et al. Arthroscopic anterior capsular reconstruction of the hip for recurrent instability. Arthrosc Tech 2015;4(6):e711–5.
42. Jacobsen S, Guth JJ, Schimoler PJ, et al. Biomechanical response to distraction of hip capsular reconstruction with human acellular dermal patch graft. Arthrosc J Arthrosc Relat Surg 2020;36(5):1337–42.
43. Scheidt M, Bhatia S, Fenoglio Z, et al. Capsular reconstruction of the hip using modified kite technique: a technical guide for efficient graft management and fixation. Arthrosc Tech 2021;10(1):e209–16.
44. Kolaczko JG, Wait T, Stevanovic O, et al. A modified "shuttle" method technique for arthroscopic hip capsular reconstruction in capsular deficiency. Arthrosc Tech 2023;12(9):e1479–85.
45. Jin T, Zhang J. Concurrent arthroscopic revision of the hip labral and anterior capsular reconstruction utilizing iliotibial band autograft. Arthrosc Tech 2025;14(5):103366. https://doi.org/10.1016/j.eats.2024.103366.
46. Meta F, Clark SC, Krych AJ, et al. Arthroscopic hip capsular reconstruction: a step-by-step guide with rectus overlay. Arthrosc Tech 2024;13(6):102982. https://doi.org/10.1016/j.eats.2024.102982.
47. DeFroda SF, Alter TD, Wichman DM, et al. Arthroscopic anchor-based hip capsular reconstruction without graft augmentation. Arthrosc Tech 2021;10(6):e1511–5.
48. Featherall J, Metz AK, Rosenthal RM, et al. Comparison of interportal and periportal capsulotomies and axial distraction resistance during hip arthroscopy: an in vivo propensity-matched cohort study. Am J Sports Med 2025;53(3):699–707.
49. Wong S, Newhouse A, Chahla J, et al. Arthroscopic treatment of hip dislocation after previous hip arthroscopy: capsular reconstruction with labral augmentation. Arthrosc Tech 2021;10(3):e867–72.
50. Byrd JWT. Hip capsular reconstruction made easy: the timing and the technique. Arthrosc Tech 2021;10(1):e73–8.
51. Kurz AZ, Memon M, Williams D, et al. Anterior capsule reconstruction of the native hip: a technique guide. Arthrosc Tech 2019;8(10):e1247–53.
52. Chahla J, Dean CS, Soares E, et al. Hip capsular reconstruction using dermal allograft. Arthrosc Tech 2016;5(2):e365–9.
53. Mameri ES, Batra AK, Kerzner B, et al. Hip capsular reconstruction with indirect head of the rectus femoris tendon. Arthrosc Tech 2023;12(4):e503–9.
54. Trindade CAC, Sawyer GA, Fukui K, et al. Arthroscopic capsule reconstruction in the hip using iliotibial band allograft. Arthrosc Tech 2015;4(1):e71–4.
55. Baha P, Burkhart TA, Getgood A, et al. Complete capsular repair restores native kinematics after interportal and T-Capsulotomy. Am J Sports Med 2019;47(6):1451–8.
56. Ekhtiari S, de Sa D, Haldane CE, et al. Hip arthroscopic capsulotomy techniques and capsular management strategies: a systematic review. Knee Surg Sports Traumatol Arthrosc Off J ESSKA 2017;25(1):9–23.
57. Philippon MJ, Michalski MP, Campbell KJ, et al. A quantitative analysis of hip capsular thickness. Knee Surg Sports Traumatol Arthrosc Off J ESSKA 2015;23(9):2548–53.
58. Telleria JJM, Lindsey DP, Giori NJ, et al. An anatomic arthroscopic description of the hip capsular ligaments for the hip arthroscopist. Arthrosc J Arthrosc Relat Surg 2011;27(5):628–36.

59. Kerzner B, Dasari SP, Khan ZA, et al. Capsular management at the time of hip arthroscopy for femoroacetabular impingement syndrome varies with geography and surgeon subspecialty training: a cross-sectional, multinational surgeon survey. Arthrosc J Arthrosc Relat Surg 2024;40(11):2695–703.e1.
60. Chambers CC, Monroe EJ, Flores SE, et al. Periportal capsulotomy: technique and outcomes for a limited capsulotomy during hip arthroscopy. Arthrosc J Arthrosc Relat Surg 2019;35(4):1120–7.
61. Klug T, Fox JD, Rosa R, et al. Patients undergoing hip arthroscopy with periportal and puncture capsulotomy demonstrate favorable outcomes at short-term follow-up: a systematic review. Arthrosc J Arthrosc Relat Surg Off Publ Arthrosc Assoc N Am Int Arthrosc Assoc 2025. https://doi.org/10.1016/j.arthro.2025.01.027. S0749-8063(25)00045-3.

Ischiofemoral Impingement: Pathophysiology, Diagnosis, and Treatment

Emmett J. Cleary, MD[a], Jacob J. Schaefer, MD[a],
Luke S. Spencer Gardner, MD[b,*]

KEYWORDS

- Ischiofemoral • Impingement • Lesser trochanterplasty • Buttock pain
- Hip arthroscopy • Hip endoscopy • Ischium

KEY POINTS

- Ischiofemoral impingement (IFI) is an under-recognized source of extra-articular hip pain characterized by pathologic narrowing of the ischiofemoral space.
- Idiopathic presentations can occur across the lifespan but are most commonly seen in middle-aged female patients due to sex-based differences in osseous morphology and age-related changes in local soft tissue structures.
- Patients present with deep buttock and groin pain exacerbated by sitting and walking that may be accompanied by mechanical snapping during the terminal stance phase of the gait cycle.
- MRI findings suggestive of IFI include decreased ischiofemoral space and quadratus femoris edema.
- Nonsurgical treatment consists of activity modification, physical therapy, gait retraining and guided injections, with generally good results. For those with persistent or recalcitrant symptoms, surgical decompression of the ischiofemoral space is recommended.

Video content accompanies this article at http://www.sportsmed.theclinics.com.

INTRODUCTION

Ischiofemoral impingement (IFI) is an extra-articular hip disorder characterized by pathologic conflict between the ischium and the lesser trochanter (LT). Dynamic impingement between the LT and ischial tuberosity results in degenerative changes

[a] Department of Orthopedic Surgery, Mayo Clinic, Rochester, MN, USA; [b] Department of Orthopedic Surgery, Mayo Clinic, Jacksonville, FL, USA
* Corresponding author. Mayo Clinic Florida, Department of Orthopedic Surgery, 4500 San Pablo Road S, Jacksonville, FL 32224.
E-mail address: Spencer-gardner.luke@mayo.edu

Clin Sports Med 45 (2026) 693–706
https://doi.org/10.1016/j.csm.2026.04.002 sportsmed.theclinics.com

Abbreviations	
IFD	ischiofemoral distance
IFI	ischiofemoral impingement
IFS	ischiofemoral space
LT	lesser trochanter
PT	physical therapy
QFS	quadratus femoris space
THA	total hip arthroplasty

in the quadratus femoris and leading to pain, snapping, and occasionally distal dysesthesias secondary to irritation or compression of the sciatic nerve.

IFI was first described in 1977 in a series of 3 patients with deep gluteal pain following total hip arthroplasty (THA).[1] The modern clinical and radiographic understanding of idiopathic IFI in the native hip was described by Patti and colleagues and Torriani and colleagues, with the authors first introducing the concept with a case report and subsequently describing a series of 12 patients presenting with deep buttock pain and characteristic findings of reduced ischiofemoral distance (IFD) and quadratus femoris edema on MRI.[2,3] In subsequent years, the body of literature on IFI has grown and has contributed to a deeper understanding of anatomic factors that contribute to the condition, and to the development of therapeutic interventions to successfully treat symptomatic IFI.

ANATOMY

The ischiofemoral space (IFS) is an anatomic interval in the deep gluteal space defined medially by the ischium and laterally by the LT and proximal femur.[4] The quadratus femoris muscle fills the space, arising from the lateral border of the ischial tuberosity, coursing laterally and proximally to insert on the quadrate tubercle and the intertrochanteric crest of the proximal femur.[5] The sciatic nerve courses posterolateral to the space on the posterior surface of the quadratus femoris, with several described configurations in relation to the piriformis.[6] The proximal hamstrings origin borders the IFS posteromedially and can be impacted in cases of severe chronic impingement; enthesopathy or avulsion of these tendons can contribute to development of IFI as well.[7,8] The IFS is measured between the lateral cortex of the ischial tuberosity and the medial cortex of the LT.[3] The quadratus femoris space (QFS) is defined as the interval between the proximal hamstring tendons and the iliopsoas insertion at the LT and represents the true anatomic space of the quadratus femoris muscle and the sciatic nerve.[3] The dimensions of the IFS are dynamic, with the interval between LT and ischium varying depending on limb position. This has been validated in cadaver studies, with the distance between the LT and ischium narrowest in 60° of external rotation; 84% of hips demonstrated mechanical contact between the LT and ischium at a mean of 29° external rotation when starting in 10° of adduction and 10° of extension.[9] Several intrinsic and extrinsic factors contribute to the pathologic narrowing of the IFS.

PATHOGENESIS AND EPIDEMIOLOGY

Narrowing of the IFS can occur primarily in the setting of anatomic variants, including coxa valga, increased femoral anteversion, decreased femoral offset, increased intertuberous distance, and increased femoral and hemipelvic anteversion.[10,11] These morphologic variants appear more commonly in female patients, likely precipitating the female predominance seen in this disorder.[12] Symptomatic IFI is more prevalent in early middle-age, suggesting extraosseous factors as well. One study noted a higher incidence of ipsilateral abductor tendinopathy in patients with IFI, suggesting that abductor weakness may cause dynamic hip adduction through the gait cycle that causes underlying anatomic abnormalities to develop into clinically symptomatic IFI.[13] Spinal pathology may also play a role, as cadaver studies have shown posterior pelvic tilt to be associated with functional narrowing of the IFS.[14]

The overall incidence is yet undefined, as symptomatic IFI appears to be a rare entity, and musculoskeletal clinicians have only recently begun to recognize and diagnose this pathology. A female predominance has been noted in reported cases, with 86% female and median age 50.8 years in one recent meta-analysis.[15]

IFI can occur secondarily due to trauma, with displacement or malunion of the medialized LT causing osseous impingement.[1] IFI has been reported as a sequela of exostosis of the LT, as in such syndromes as multiple hereditary exostosis.[16,17] Space-occupying lesions have also been implicated.[18] IFI has also been reported in the setting of proximal hamstring dysfunction after ischial apophyseal avulsion malunion, with good results for open resection and proximal hamstring repair reported in a small series of cases.[7,8]

IFI can occur iatrogenically after arthroplasty, valgus-producing or derotational femoral osteotomy, or periacetabular osteotomy, due to reduction in offset or alterations in femoral or hemipelvic version.[1,19]

A recent investigation using validated morphometric parameters to assess gait kinematics found notable sexual dimorphism in pelvic anatomy, likely related to obstetric requirements, that account for most of the sex-based difference in ischiofemoral clearance.[11] While female pelvic width is roughly equal to that of males, interischial distance was higher in female hips, and femoral offset is notably higher in male hips. The authors also observed an association with interspinous distance normalized to pelvic width, introducing an ischial spine ratio which functions as a measure of hemipelvic version. Low ischial-spine ratio suggests retroversion that would comparatively medialize the ischial tuberosity, improving clearance of the LT, whereas a higher ischial spine ratio—connoting hemipelvic anteversion and lateralization of the ischial tuberosity—increases the likelihood of anatomic conflict and IFI.[11]

CLINICAL EVALUATION

Patients with IFI usually present with deep gluteal pain that worsens in the terminal extension phase of the gait cycle. Pain is often exacerbated by sitting on the affected region, and patients may offload the affected side by leaning to the unaffected side while in the seated position. Buttock pain may be accompanied by deep groin pain. This presentation may mimic osteoarthritis, acetabular labral tears, acetabular dysplasia, lumbar radiculopathy, proximal hamstring tendinopathy/tearing, sacroiliac pain, and piriformis syndrome.[20] Careful examination is necessary to delineate IFI from these other etiologies.

Physical examination of the painful hip should begin with gait assessment. Patients with IFI may walk with short steps to avoid long strides, as the IFS is narrowed in hip extension. Buttock and groin pain and mechanical snapping can often be replicated by the *long stride test* where the patient is instructed to exaggerate a long step forward with the unaffected hip, maximally extending the painful side. Reported sensitivity is 94% with specificity 85%.[21] (Video 1).

The affected extremity can then be examined in the seated position, assessing hip range of motion in 90° of flexion. The ischium and IFS can be palpated with the patient seated. Pain lateral to the ischium is suggestive of IFI, pain over the ischium may be associated with proximal hamstrings tendinopathy, and pain medial to the ischium may be suggestive of extraosseous etiologies such as pudendal neuralgia.[22] Resisted knee flexion can be used to determine the extent of symptomatic proximal hamstrings pain.

The limb should then be examined in the supine position, first with palpation of the inguinal region to rule out extra-articular causes of groin pain. The hip joint range of motion should be assessed, and provocative maneuvers such as the Stinchfield test and flexion adduction and internal rotation tests can help differentiate intra-articular sources. Resisted hip adduction and concomitant sit up test can be used to assess for sports hernia/athletic pubalgia. A thorough strength exam should be performed of all lower extremity myotomes, especially in the case of any symptoms of sciatica.

The patient should then be positioned in the lateral decubitus position, lying on the unaffected side. The examiner should palpate the greater trochanter, ischial tuberosity, deep gluteal space including the expected course of the piriformis, and sacroiliac joint, assessing for pain in each area. Palpation of the IFS between the greater trochanter and the ischium may elicit pain, suggesting the presence of IFI. Passive internal rotation in extension and resisted external rotation can be used to assess pathology related to piriformis syndrome. The hip is then passively extended, adducted, and externally rotated. This *IFI test* is positive if it reproduces symptoms, with reported sensitivity of 82% and specificity 85%.[21] Limited external rotation, especially in the setting of increased femoral or combined femoral and acetabular version, is also associated with posterior extra-articular osseous impingement as in IFI.[10]

RADIOGRAPHIC EVALUATION

Characteristic imaging findings are integral to make the diagnosis of symptomatic IFI. Radiographs should be obtained for any patient presenting with a persistently painful hip. In most cases of IFI these will be grossly normal, though there can be anatomic variants including coxa valga that may predispose patients to reduced IFD and symptomatic IFI. Osseous projections from the LT or the ischium will likewise decrease the available volume of the IFS (**Fig. 1**A–C). Long-leg radiographs showed a significant association between valgus knee alignment and narrow IFD; however, this imaging exam is not routinely obtained in the evaluation of IFI.[23]

MRI remains the gold standard for diagnosis of IFI in the likely event that plain radiographs are nondiagnostic. MRI has the advantage of quantifying IFD, IFS, and QFS on

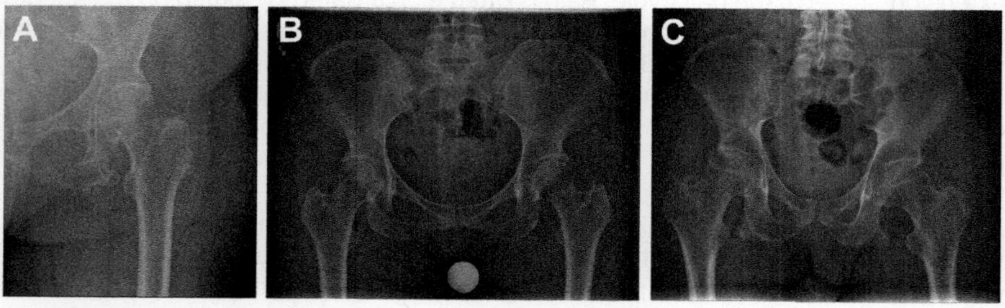

Fig. 1. (*A*) Anteroposterior (AP) radiograph of a left hip in a patient with symptomatic IFI secondary to coxa valga and enthesopathy of the proximal hamstrings (*B*) AP pelvis radiograph of a patient with IFI secondary to enthesopathy of the right lesser trochanter (*C*) AP pelvis radiograph of a patient with IFI secondary to enthesopathy of the bilateral ischial tuberosities.

axial sequences, as it can best characterize soft tissue mass at the LT and proximal hamstring origin.[5] MRI also has the ability to evaluate the quadratus femoris for edema and intrasubstance tear to suggest dynamic impingement.[24] Fatty infiltration of the quadratus femoris muscle belly and hamstring tendon area have both been associated with symptomatic IFI.[25] Further evaluation of the sciatic nerve is also helpful to explain symptoms that may be referred distally.[24] In cases of chromic, severe IFI, marrow edema or subcortical cysts may be seen in the ischium or LT.[26] (**Fig. 2**A–C).

With regard to quantitative parameters of the IFS and QFS, an IF space less than or equal to 15 mm demonstrates a sensitivity of 77%, specificity of 81%, and an overall accuracy of 78% for identifying narrowing, and a QFS less than or equal to 10 mm demonstrating a sensitivity of 78%, a specificity of 74%, and an overall accuracy of 77% for identifying narrowing.[15]

It is critical to recognize that hip positioning can influence the above measurements. External rotation of the hip can narrow the ischiofemoral (IF) interval.[26,27] Dynamic MRI studies demonstrated asymmetric decrease in IFS and QFS with maximal external rotation, causing IFS reduction of 59% in narrowed hips versus 41% in control hips, and QFS decreased 71% in narrowed hips versus 50% in control hips. These differences were not apparent in neutral rotation.[28] In a small study of asymptomatic patients, dynamic fluoroscopy demonstrated significant reductions in IFS during external rotation, extension, and gait that compared to those measured on supine MRI, prompting the authors to advocate for extension, adduction, and external rotation of the affected hip during clinical and radiologic evaluation.[29] A study comparing standardized positioning for MRI to nonstandardized positioning of the same hip from outside institution found 19% of those with symptomatic IFI were categorized as normal in the nonstandardized MRI, most commonly due to hip flexion and rotation.[30]

Finally, evaluation of axial alignment with either magnetic ressonance (MR) of computed tomography (CT) imaging is recommended to assess contributions from abnormal femoral anteversion. Though rarely the predominant feature, sciatic nerve dysesthesias may be present and, in such cases, lumbar imaging and electromyography may be warranted.[31]

NONSURGICAL MANAGEMENT

After establishing the diagnosis of IFI, targeted nonsurgical treatment is initiated. Activity modification begins with gait retraining to promote shortening of the stride length to avoid impingement in terminal extension. Cushions may be used to offload the IFS

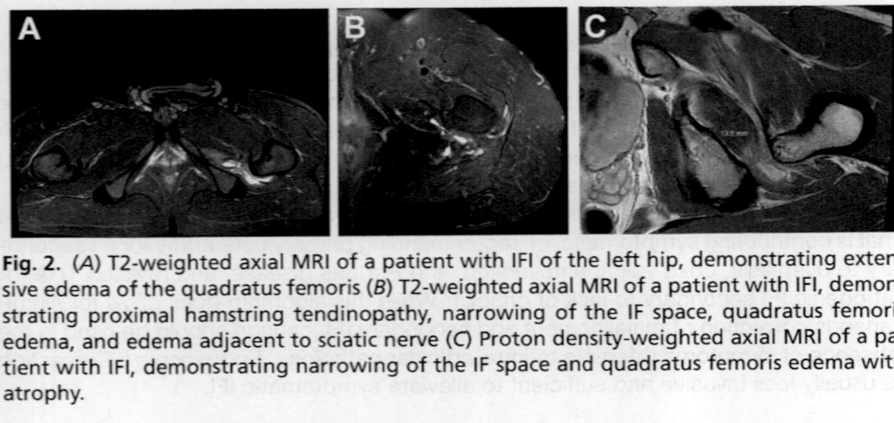

Fig. 2. (*A*) T2-weighted axial MRI of a patient with IFI of the left hip, demonstrating extensive edema of the quadratus femoris (*B*) T2-weighted axial MRI of a patient with IFI, demonstrating proximal hamstring tendinopathy, narrowing of the IF space, quadratus femoris edema, and edema adjacent to sciatic nerve (*C*) Proton density-weighted axial MRI of a patient with IFI, demonstrating narrowing of the IF space and quadratus femoris edema with atrophy.

when sitting on hard surfaces. Anti-inflammatory medications may alleviate pain, and a course of physical therapy (PT) should be prescribed. Specific PT protocols are not well-described, though there is a biomechanical basis for abductor strengthening as a means to prevent dynamic adduction that brings the hip into positions of ischiofemoral conflict, and this should be the functional goal of therapy in conjunction with modalities for symptomatic treatment.[13] Case reports document improvement with strengthening of the abductors and external rotators, as well as with heat, ultrasound, stretching, kinesiotaping, dry needling, and transcutaneous electrical nerve stimulation.[32,33] Ultrasound or CT-guided injections are integral in the diagnostic workup and are used to differentiate symptomatic IFI from other sources of pain affecting the deep gluteal space, as well as for providing symptomatic relief.[34]

SURGICAL MANAGEMENT

If symptoms persist despite a dedicated course of nonsurgical treatment, surgery should be considered. The planned procedure should address the structural driver of the impingement while minimizing soft tissue injury and risks to surrounding neurovascular structures. Given the varied etiologies contributing to the diagnosis of IFI, several surgical treatment options have been described and successfully implemented.

Early reports advocated for open resection of the LT, ischial tuberosity, or both.[35–37] Good results have been described, but there is significant morbidity associated with open approaches to the IFS. Some authors advocate for performing limited sciatic neurolysis, proximal hamstring debridement and reattachment, and decompressive resection of the LT to address multiple etiologies and pain drivers, however complications including hematoma and sciatic nerve injury have been reported.[38,39]

Varus-producing, lateralizing, and derotational osteotomies have the advantage of being able to correct version and severe coxa valga, and there are case reports of good results for isolated IFI.[40–42] Varus-producing osteotomies about the knee have also been suggested, though currently this is theoretic.[23]

Endoscopy has gained popularity as a minimally invasive technique for addressing IFI. First reported in 2014 by Safran, most authors advocate for anteriorly based techniques with the hip externally rotated in the supine position, allowing endoscopic resection with minimal risk to the sciatic nerve.[43–45] Alternately, some authors recommend posteriorly based portals to perform sciatic nerve decompression and preserve the anterior fibers of the iliopsoas.[43,46,47] An anteriorly based technique with reattachment of the iliopsoas to the resected LT footprint has also been described.[45]

In patients with residual, persistent, or iatrogenic IFI after THA, endoscopic resection of the LT can be considered as a less invasive option compared to revision surgery. If there is concern that LT osteoplasty would be inadequate, or if revision arthroplasty would be otherwise indicated in the setting of instability, or if there are other drivers such as prosthetic or greater trochanteric impingement, revision THA can be used with a goal of adding offset, correcting any version abnormalities, and allowing open bony resection as needed.

Some authors advocate for structural correction of any underlying anatomic variant that is contributing symptomatic IFI, recommending primary osteotomy for IFI secondary to dysplasia, coxa valga, anteversion, and Perthes disease, and revision THA for iatrogenic IFI secondary to lack of offset.[48] While this algorithm does allow for simultaneous correction of malalignment and secondary IFI, caution should be used in the absence of symptoms referable to intra-articular pathology. Endoscopic LT resection is usually less invasive and sufficient to alleviate symptomatic IFI.

There are reports of patients with recalcitrant IFI being indicated for THA in the absence of significant osteoarthritis—the authors do not recommend such management for isolated IFI without intra-articular pathology supporting conversion to THA.

PREFERRED SURGICAL TECHNIQUE

The authors recommend endoscopic decompression of the IFS by isolated resection of the LT using the technique described by Goodwin and colleagues[49] This method reliably achieves safe and predictable decompression of the IFS with minimal complications in experienced hands.

After appropriate preoperative evaluation, medical optimization, and informed consent, the patient is taken to the operating room. The authors prefer supine positioning on a distraction table (Smith & Nephew) without the perineal post, to control the leg, and maximize fluoroscopic visualization. However, a radiolucent operating room table would also suffice. Anesthesia is induced, antibiotics are administered, and the affected anterolateral hip and thigh are sterilely prepped and draped from the iliac crest to the knee. A straight line is drawn from the anterosuperior iliac spine to the proximal pole of the patella, deemed as the safe line to reference while establishing portals. Care should be taken to make portals lateral to this *safe line* to minimize the risk to neurovascular structures.

Using fluoroscopic guidance, the level of the LT is identified. Two endoscopic portals are established greater than 2 to 3 cm lateral to the *safe line*. Portals should be placed approximately 5 cm apart, with convergent trajectory toward the level of the LT. The Seldinger technique is used to establish the viewing portal proximally, followed by the working portal distally under fluoroscopic guidance. Tactile feedback on the LT is also used when establishing portals. The arthroscopic fluid pump pressure is kept low (<40 mm Hg) to minimize the risk of fluid extravasation and abdominal compartment syndrome.[50,51] The overlying iliopsoas muscle fibers are cleared from the surface of the LT with radiofrequency ablation. Once visualization of the LT is established and confirmed with fluoroscopy, the hip is flexed and externally rotated to bring the LT in to view. The iliopsoas tendon is then released under direct visualization using radiofrequency ablation. The LT is then burred down to the contour of the medial femoral subtrochanteric cortex using a 5.5 mm bur. The hip is repositioned as needed to aid in visualization and ensure complete resection of the bony prominence. Fluoroscopic imaging is then used to confirm that the ischiofemoral interval is radiographically widened (**Fig. 3**A–D). At the conclusion of the case, care should be taken to ensure adequate hemostasis as there are rare reports of significant hematoma formation related to pseudoaneurysm of branches of the femoral circumflex vessels.[52] (Video 2) Postoperatively, heterotopic ossification prophylaxis is initiated with a course of nonsteroidal anti-inflammatories. Patients are allowed to bear weight as tolerated and are instructed to avoid repetitive hip flexion for 4 to 6 weeks.

Complications are rare, though several have been described that are uncommon in hip arthroscopy.[39] Endoscopy around the hip that violates the iliopsoas sheath runs the risk of retroperitoneal fluid extravasation and secondary abdominal compartment syndrome, a rare but catastrophic complication that has been reported.[50,51] As previously stated, the endoscopic pump pressure is kept low during the case to prevent fluid extravasation, and the patient's core body temperature is carefully monitored. Vascular complications can also occur—the authors are aware of at least 3 cases of medial femoral circumflex artery pseudoaneurysm requiring angioembolization.[52] The attendant iliopsoas release is generally well-tolerated; there is a small but measurable decrement in seated hip flexion strength (19%)

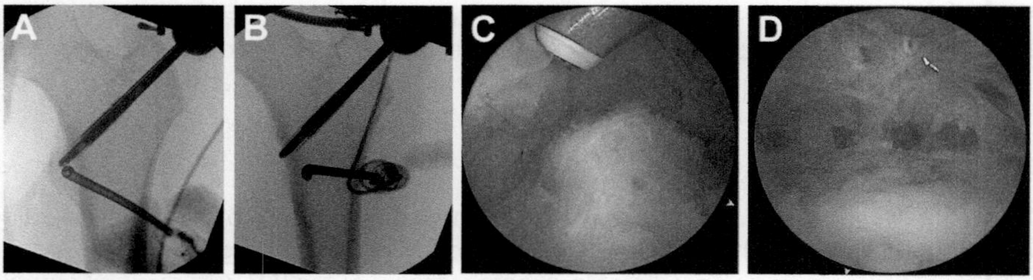

Fig. 3. (*A*) Intraoperative AP fluoroscopic image of the left hip in a patient with IFI demonstrating localization of endoscopic instruments before resection of the lesser trochanter (*B*) Intraoperative AP fluoroscopic image of the same left hip demonstrating postoperative changes following endoscopic resection of the lesser trochanter (*C*) Endoscopic view of the lesser trochanter preresection. Viewing right hip anterior to posterior, medial top, lateral bottom, proximal left and distal right, arthroscopic radiofrequency wand visualized retracting the psoas tendon after release (*D*) Endoscopic view of the lesser trochanter postresection. Viewing right hip anterior to posterior, medial top, lateral bottom, proximal left and distal right, arthroscopic shaver seen top right retracting the adjacent psoas bursa.

and cross-sectional area of the released psoas muscle belly on postoperative MRI (25%), but this has not translated into clinically meaningful weakness and patient reported outcomes following arthroscopic or endoscopic release have been routinely satisfactory.[53] (Video 3).

DISCUSSION

Although our understanding of IFI continues to grow, there remains a relative paucity of evidence to guide the optimal nonoperative and surgical management strategies as well as the indications for different interventions. Clinical outcomes have been reported in relatively small series, and the authors are aware of no high-level evidence comparing surgical with nonoperative management or results between different surgical interventions.

Early case reports of idiopathic or primary IFI demonstrated reasonable response to non-steroidal anti-inflammatory drugs (NSAIDs), activity modification, and rest, suggesting an inflammatory component to symptomatic flares.[2,7,54,55] Targeted injections, including corticosteroid, botulinum, and prolotherapy have likewise been reported efficacious in small series.[56–58]

In addition to conservative management with NSAIDs, rest, physiotherapy, and injections, there have been several case reports and small series describing the open surgical treatment of IFI. Early case reports of open resection of the LT, ischium, and congenital ischial exostosis by both anterior and posterior approaches were associated with symptomatic improvement and uncomplicated recovery.[16,35,37] Ganz and colleagues described a small series of 8 patients treated successfully via LT advancement for IFI secondary to Perthes and *Perthes-like* conditions.[36] Lerch and colleagues reported excellent midterm results of femoral subtrochanteric derotational osteotomy for IFI in a series of 23 patients with mean of 4-year follow-up, with subjective hip satisfaction increasing 24% to 84%, and 80% of patients reporting they would undergo surgery again.[42] These results must be interpreted with caution; however, as all but one of these patients underwent concomitant surgical hip dislocation with cam resection and labral treatment. Palma and colleagues reported a good result treating a patient with bilateral IFI in the setting of increased anteversion with staged derotational subtrochanteric osteotomies.[41]

Continued innovation among arthroscopic hip preservation surgeons, and the desire to avoid the morbidity associated with open approaches and femoral osteotomies, has led to the development of endoscopic techniques. Safran and Ryu described the first endoscopic IFI treatment in a case report, reporting durable symptomatic relief 2 years after resection of the LT using an arthroscopic bur.[43] Jo and O'Donnell reported a similar case the following year, with durable symptomatic relief after endoscopic resection of the LT via an anterior approach.[44] In 2015, Hatem and colleagues subsequently reported excellent 2-year results in a series of 5 patients treated with endoscopic LT resection via posteriorly based portals, with mean mHHS improving from 51.3 to 94.2, mean VAS-pain decreasing 6.6 to 1.0, 60% return to sports, and negative long stride and IFI testing in all patients.[47] Proponents of posteriorly based endoscopy highlight the desire to avoid vascular injury and preserve the iliopsoas insertion. Three of the 5 patients in this study underwent concomitant arthroscopy for intra-articular pathology, however, and these results must be interpreted in this light.[47] In 2016, Wilson and Keene reported excellent 6-month and 12-month outcomes in a series of 7 patients undergoing anteriorly based endoscopic LT resection and iliopsoas tenotomy for symptomatic IFI with positive response to image-guided IFS injections.[59] Postoperative modified harris hip score (mHHS) scores averaged 86 and 91 at 6-month and 12-month respectively, up from an average of 43 preoperatively.[59] No hip flexion weakness was appreciated on postoperative manual muscle strength testing. However, these results are also confounded by the fact that 4 of 7 patients underwent concomitant arthroscopy for articular pathology.[59] Marquez and colleagues published a series of 13 female patients, mean age 40.2 years, who underwent isolated endoscopic LT resection with similar improvements in mHHS and VAS-pain at 10-month follow-up.[60]

IFI can be a challenging diagnosis to make in isolation. The clinical picture may be obscured more so in the setting of concomitant hip osteoarthritis, or in cases of IFI post–hip arthroplasty. IFI was first described by Johnson in 1977 in a small series of patients presenting with residual pain and mechanical symptoms after otherwise successful THA.[1] Just as in the prearthritic hip, surgeons should be aware that coexisting conditions such as IFI may be present in addition to hip osteoarthritis. While end-stage osteoarthritis of the hip may complicate the clinical diagnosis of comorbid IFI, careful history and exam can elucidate the presence of symptoms that may be attributable to IFI. Targeted injections may also be helpful in differentiating whether symptoms are related to the joint or the IFS.

Despite the demonstrated utility of MRI in the diagnosis of IFI, the authors do not advocate for its routine use in the evaluation of the arthritic hip, unless symptoms clearly suggestive of IFI are present. Hip surgeons should be alert for a narrow ischiofemoral interval on AP radiographs, the presence of coxa valga, or symptomatic enthesophytes or sclerosis of the LT or ischial tuberosity. Heightened suspicion preoperatively allows the treating surgeon the opportunity to ensure adequate offset and version to achieve a stable prosthesis while avoiding persistent or recurrent IFI.

There have been isolated reports of surgeons indicating patients for THA to treat IFI in the absence of radiographically or clinically apparent articular hip pathology. The authors do not recommend this treatment approach, as despite the excellent long-term results of THA, isolated IFI can be treated effectively with less invasive, joint-sparing procedures.

During THA, reduction in offset should be avoided, as in addition to potentially compromising stability, one risks precipitating iatrogenic IFI. Some authors have argued high-offset femoral components as a risk factor for posterior bony impingement in CT models, though this has not been demonstrated in vivo.[61] Attention should likewise be paid to restoration of femoral component version to minimize the risk of iatrogenic IFI. CT and MRI-based studies have shown that postoperative femoral anteversion, especially increased anteversion from the preoperative state, is associated with development of IFI postoperatively.[19,62,63] Modular diaphyseal-engaging, or cone-body stems can be used to achieve optimal impingement-free version in the setting of significant proximal femoral deformity. The authors do not routinely perform osteoplasty of the LT or ischial tuberosity during primary or revision hip arthroplasty, as attention to restoration of adequate offset and anteversion is usually sufficient to achieve a stable, impingement-free hip.

In evaluating the painful THA, IFI should be considered only after excluding more common causes of failure such of infection, metallosis, component impingement, or loosening. Quadratus femoris edema on post-THA MRI is nondiagnostic as this finding may be related to postsurgical changes particularly after a posterior approach.[64] Correlation of IFS and QFS between plain radiographs and MRI is limited by rotation and technique.[64] Image-guided IFS space injections can be especially helpful as a diagnostic tool in this setting. As noted above, revision surgery should be reserved to patients with significant pain and debility recalcitrant to a dedicated course of nonoperative management. In the absence of gross instability or component malposition, the authors prefer endoscopic LT osteoplasty over revision arthroplasty.

SUMMARY

IFI is a rare but increasingly recognized extra-articular hip disorder characterized by pathologic compression of the quadratus femoris and occasionally the sciatic nerve between the ischium and LT. Patients present with deep buttock and groin pain exacerbated by hip extension, adduction, and external rotation; some also report mechanical symptoms and neurologic symptoms in the sciatic distribution. Characteristic imaging findings include narrowing of the IFS and quadratus femoris edema on axial MRI. Initial treatment consists of activity modification, NSAIDs, PT emphasizing gait retraining and abductor strengthening, and image-guided IFS injections. In patients with recalcitrant symptoms, surgical treatment should be used to address the underlying pathologic factors contributing to IFI. Endoscopic LT osteoplasty is the author's preferred surgical treatment for the majority of cases, with excellent short-term and midterm results and a low rate of complication or treatment failure.

CLINICS CARE POINTS

- Patients with ischiofemoral impingement (IFI) present with buttock and groin pain and may report mechanical symptoms during the gait cycle when the affected hip is in terminal extension.
- Clinicians should maintain a high index of suspicion in the setting of coxa valga, increased femoral anteversion, and in cases of bony prominences or enthesopathy emanating from the lesser trochanter or the ischium.
- Pathognomonic MRI findings include narrowing of the ischiofemoral space less than 15 mm on axial sequences, and quadratus femoris edema/atrophy.
- IFI is dynamic and positional. Limb position during radiographs and MRI should be standardized, as internal rotation or flexion of the hip can falsely increase the ischiofemoral distance.
- Image-guided anesthetic and corticosteroid injection are useful to differentiate IFI from other causes of hip and buttock pain and often confers lasting symptomatic benefit.
- Endoscopic management, via resection of the lesser trochanter offers predictable symptomatic improvement in the hands of experienced surgeons. Care must be taken to

avoid iatrogenic neurovascular injury, hematoma formation, or intra-abdominal fluid extravasation, using low pump pressures and core temperature monitoring.

- Iatrogenic IFI should be avoided in the setting of arthroplasty and femoral or pelvic osteotomy by careful attention to appropriate component positioning, offset, and version. Surgeons should suspect IFI as a cause of pain after total hip arthroplasty only when infection, loosening, instability, and iliopsoas impingement have been ruled out.

DISCLOSURE

Dr L.S. Spencer-Gardner is a consultant for Smith and Nephew and Medacta, USA. He receives royalties from Medacta, USA.

SUPPLEMENTARY DATA

Supplementary data related to this article can be found online at https://doi.org/10.1016/j.csm.2026.04.002.

REFERENCES

1. Johnson KA. Impingement of the lesser trochanter on the ischial ramus after total hip arthroplasty. Report of three cases. J Bone Joint Surg Am 1977;59(2):268–9.
2. Patti JW, Ouellette H, Bredella MA, et al. Impingement of lesser trochanter on ischium as a potential cause for hip pain. Skelet Radiol 2008;37(10):939–41.
3. Torriani M, Souto SCL, Thomas BJ, et al. Ischiofemoral impingement syndrome: an entity with hip pain and abnormalities of the quadratus femoris muscle. AJR Am J Roentgenol 2009;193(1):186–90.
4. Martin HD PI, Hatem MA. Deep gluteal syndrome. Hip arthroscopy and hip joint preservation surgery. Springer; 2014. p. 1–30.
5. Kassarjian A, Tomas X, Cerezal L, et al. MRI of the quadratus femoris muscle: anatomic considerations and pathologic lesions. AJR Am J Roentgenol 2011; 197(1):170–4.
6. Natsis K, Totlis T, Konstantinidis GA, et al. Anatomical variations between the sciatic nerve and the piriformis muscle: a contribution to surgical anatomy in Piriformis syndrome. Surg Radiol Anat 2014;36(3):273–80.
7. Hayat Z, Konan S, Pollock R. Ischiofemoral impingement resulting from a chronic avulsion injury of the hamstrings. BMJ Case Rep 2014;2014.
8. Spencer-Gardner L, Bedi A, Stuart MJ, et al. Ischiofemoral impingement and hamstring dysfunction as a potential pain generator after ischial tuberosity apophyseal fracture non-union/malunion. Knee Surg Sports Traumatol Arthrosc 2017;25(1):55–61.
9. Kivlan BR, Martin RL, Martin HD. Ischiofemoral impingement: defining the lesser trochanter-ischial space. Knee Surg Sports Traumatol Arthrosc 2017;25(1):72–6.
10. Boschung A, Antioco T, Steppacher SD, et al. Limited external rotation and hip extension due to posterior extra-articular ischiofemoral hip impingement in female patients with increased femoral anteversion: implications for sports, sexual, and daily activities. Am J Sports Med 2023;51(4):1015–23.
11. Audenaert EA, Duquesne K, De Roeck J, et al. Ischiofemoral impingement: the evolutionary cost of pelvic obstetric adaptation. J Hip Preserv Surg 2020;7(4): 677–87.
12. Stafford GH, Villar RN. Ischiofemoral impingement. J Bone Joint Surg Br 2011;93-(10):1300–2.

13. Kheterpal AB, Harvey JP, Husseini JS, et al. Hip abductor tears in ischiofemoral impingement. Skelet Radiol 2020;49(11):1747–52.
14. Spencer-Gardner L, Nunley B, Gómez-Hoyos J, et al. Sagittal pelvic tilt directly influences the ischiofemoral space: a cadaveric study. Orthopedics 2024;47(3):167–71.
15. Singer AD, Subhawong TK, Jose J, et al. Ischiofemoral impingement syndrome: a meta-analysis. Skelet Radiol 2015;44(6):831–7.
16. Viala P, Vanel D, Larbi A, et al. Bilateral ischiofemoral impingement in a patient with hereditary multiple exostoses. Skelet Radiol 2012;41(12):1637–40.
17. Elnaggar A, Abraham R, Hasanain S, et al. Incidental finding of hereditary multiple osteochondroma causing ischiofemoral impingement. BMJ Case Rep 2021;14(9).
18. Papoutsi D, Daniels J, Mistry A, et al. Ischiofemoral impingement due to a lipoma of the ischiofemoral space. BMJ Case Rep 2016;2016.
19. Fischer T, Stern C, Fritz B, et al. MRI findings of ischiofemoral impingement after total hip arthroplasty are associated with increased femoral antetorsion. Acta Radiol 2022;63(7):948–57.
20. Gonzalez-Lomas G. Deep gluteal pain in orthopaedics: a challenging diagnosis. J Am Acad Orthop Surg 2021;29(24):e1282–90.
21. Martin HD, Khoury A, Schröder R, et al. Ischiofemoral impingement and hamstring syndrome as causes of posterior hip pain: where do we go next? Clin Sports Med 2016;35(3):469–86.
22. Gómez-Hoyos J, Martin RL, Martin HD. Current concepts review: evaluation and management of posterior hip pain. J Am Acad Orthop Surg 2018;26(17):597–609.
23. Ahmad SS, Kerber V, Konrads C, et al. The ischiofemoral space of the hip is influenced by the frontal knee alignment. Knee Surg Sports Traumatol Arthrosc 2021;29(8):2446–52.
24. Taneja AK, Bredella MA, Torriani M. Ischiofemoral impingement. Magn Reson Imag Clin N Am 2013;21(1):65–73.
25. Tosun O, Algin O, Yalcin N, et al. Ischiofemoral impingement: evaluation with new MRI parameters and assessment of their reliability. Skelet Radiol 2012;41(5):575–87.
26. Torriani M. Ischiofemoral impingement syndrome in 2024: updated concepts and imaging methods. Magn Reson Imag Clin N Am 2025;33(1):63–73.
27. Lerch TD, Huber FA, Bredella MA, et al. MRI 3D simulation of hip motion in female patients with and without ischiofemoral impingement. Skelet Radiol 2024;53(1):67–73.
28. Vicentini JRT, Martinez-Salazar EL, Simeone FJ, et al. Kinematic MRI of ischiofemoral impingement. Skelet Radiol 2021;50(1):97–106.
29. Atkins PR, Fiorentino NM, Aoki SK, et al. In vivo measurements of the ischiofemoral space in recreationally active participants during dynamic activities: a high-speed dual fluoroscopy study. Am J Sports Med 2017;45(12):2901–10.
30. Hatem M, Martin RL, Nimmons SJ, et al. Frequency of ischiofemoral space discrepancy when comparing magnetic resonance images of distinct institutions for the same patient. SAVE Proc 2020;34(2):242–6.
31. Hotait M, Makki A, Sawaya R. Ischiofemoral impingement syndrome: a case report redefining this condition. Neurosurg Rev 2016;39(4):707–9.
32. Ata AM, Yavuz H, Kaymak B, et al. Ischiofemoral impingement revisited: what physiatrists need to know in short. Am J Phys Med Rehabil 2014;93(12):1104.
33. Mohammed FA, Alotaibi AN, Hamdi MA, et al. Physical therapy management of ischiofemoral impingement syndrome: a case report. World J Clin Cases 2025;13(20):105606.

34. Heimann AF, Wagner M, Vavron P, et al. CT-guided infiltration of the ischiofemoral space in young patients with ischiofemoral impingement is an effective diagnostic tool. Insights Imaging 2024;15(1):235.
35. Ali AM, Whitwell D, Ostlere SJ. Case report: imaging and surgical treatment of a snapping hip due to ischiofemoral impingement. Skelet Radiol 2011;40(5):653–6.
36. Ganz R, Slongo T, Turchetto L, et al. The lesser trochanter as a cause of hip impingement: pathophysiology and treatment options. Hip Int 2013;23(Suppl 9):S35–41.
37. Truong WH, Murnaghan ML, Hopyan S, et al. Ischioplasty for femoroischial impingement: a case report. JBJS Case Connect 2012;2(3):e51.
38. Curley AJ, Setliff JC, Greiner JJ, et al. Comprehensive open management of buttock/ischiofemoral symptoms: the COMBIS procedure for posterior hip pain. Video J Sports Med 2022;2(6):26350254221129627.
39. Aguilera-Bohórquez B, Pacheco J, Castillo L, et al. Complications of hip endoscopy in the treatment of subgluteal space pathologies. Arthroscopy 2021;37(7): 2152–61.
40. Suren C, Burgkart R, Banke IJ, et al. [Surgical therapy of ischiofemoral impingement by lateralizing intertrochanteric osteotomy]. Operat Orthop Traumatol 2018; 30(2):98–110.
41. Palma I, Nave A, Torres T, et al. Minimally invasive solutions for ischiofemoral impingement: case analysis and evolving surgical strategies. J Hip Preserv Surg 2025;12(2):144–9.
42. Lerch TD, Schmaranzer F, Steppacher SD, et al. Most of patients with femoral derotation osteotomy for posterior extraarticular hip impingement and high femoral version would do surgery again. Hip Int 2022;32(2):253–64.
43. Safran M, Ryu J. Ischiofemoral impingement of the hip: a novel approach to treatment. Knee Surg Sports Traumatol Arthrosc 2014;22(4):781–5.
44. Jo S, O'Donnell JM. Endoscopic lesser trochanter resection for treatment of ischiofemoral impingement. J Hip Preserv Surg 2015;2(2):184–9.
45. Corrales R, Mediavilla I, Margalet E, et al. Endoscopic lesser trochanter resection with refixation of the iliopsoas tendon for treatment of ischiofemoral impingement. Arthrosc Tech 2018;7(4):e321–5.
46. Howse EA, Mannava S, Tamam C, et al. Ischiofemoral space decompression through posterolateral approach: cutting block technique. Arthrosc Tech 2014; 3(6):e661–5.
47. Hatem MA, Palmer IJ, Martin HD. Diagnosis and 2-year outcomes of endoscopic treatment for ischiofemoral impingement. Arthroscopy 2015;31(2):239–46.
48. Gollwitzer H, Banke IJ, Schauwecker J, et al. How to address ischiofemoral impingement? Treatment algorithm and review of the literature. J Hip Preserv Surg 2017;4(4):289–98.
49. Goodwin JA, Chhabra A, Patel KA, et al. Lesser trochanter osteoplasty for ischiofemoral impingement. Arthrosc Tech 2017;6(5):e1755–60.
50. Shakuo T, Bito K, Yasuda S, et al. Abdominal compartment syndrome during hip arthroscopy for an acetabular fracture: a case report. JA Clin Rep 2017;3(1):24.
51. Hinzpeter J, Barrientos C, Barahona M, et al. Fluid extravasation related to hip arthroscopy: a prospective computed tomography-based study. Orthop J Sports Med 2015;3(3):2325967115573222.
52. Nakano N, Lisenda L, Khanduja V. Pseudoaneurysm of a branch of the femoral circumflex artery as a complication of revision arthroscopic release of the iliopsoas tendon. SICOT J 2017;3:26.

53. Brandenburg JB, Kapron AL, Wylie JD, et al. The functional and structural outcomes of arthroscopic iliopsoas release. Am J Sports Med 2016;44(5):1286–91.
54. Tosun Ö, Çay N, Bozkurt M, et al. Ischiofemoral impingement in an 11-year-old girl. Diagn Interv Radiol 2012;18(6):571–3.
55. Lee S, Kim I, Lee SM, et al. Ischiofemoral impingement syndrome. Ann Rehabil Med 2013;37(1):143–6.
56. Kim WJ, Shin HY, Koo GH, et al. Ultrasound-guided prolotherapy with polydeoxyribonucleotide sodium in ischiofemoral impingement syndrome. Pain Pract 2014;14(7):649–55.
57. Backer MW, Lee KS, Blankenbaker DG, et al. Correlation of ultrasound-guided corticosteroid injection of the quadratus femoris with MRI findings of ischiofemoral impingement. AJR Am J Roentgenol 2014;203(3):589–93.
58. Chen YT, Jenkins KM. Ultrasound finding of ischiofemoral impingement syndrome and novel treatment with botulinum toxin chemodenervation: a case report. Pm r 2018;10(6):665–70.
59. Wilson MD, Keene JS. Treatment of ischiofemoral impingement: results of diagnostic injections and arthroscopic resection of the lesser trochanter. J Hip Preserv Surg 2016;3(2):146–53.
60. Marquez WH, Carro LP, Bohorquez BA, et al. Ischiofemoral impingement: from anatomy to endoscopic decompression. JAAOS 2017;25(10):724.
61. Shoji T, Yamasaki T, Izumi S, et al. Factors affecting the potential for posterior bony impingement after total hip arthroplasty. Bone Joint J 2017;99-b(9):1140–6.
62. Marth AA, Goller SS, Sutter R. Femoral anteversion change is associated with ischiofemoral impingement after total hip arthroplasty: a retrospective CT evaluation. Eur Radiol 2024;34(6):3529–37.
63. Shozen H, Shoji T, Ueki S, et al. Analysis of posterior hip joint impingement about developmental dysplasia of the hip after total hip arthroplasty. Clin Biomech 2025;122:106422.
64. Oliveira AL, Azevedo DC, Eajazi A, et al. Assessment of total hip arthroplasty as a predisposing factor for ischiofemoral impingement. Skelet Radiol 2015;44(12):1755–60.

Iliopsoas Impingement and the Post-Total Hip Arthroplasty Hip

Alex R. Oles, MD, PhD[a], John J. Kelly, MD[a], Bruce A. Levy, MD[b], Mario Hevesi, MD, PhD[a,*]

KEYWORDS

- Iliopsoas impingement • Total hip arthroplasty • Arthroscopic iliopsoas tenotomy
- Fractional lengthening • Postoperative hip pain • Hip flexor pathology

KEY POINTS

- Iliopsoas impingement is an underrecognized cause of persistent groin pain after total hip arthroplasty.
- Etiologies include acetabular cup prominence, collared femoral stems, altered femoral version, and tendon-specific factors.
- Diagnosis requires careful clinical assessment, exclusion of other causes of pain, and targeted imaging, with ultrasound offering both diagnostic and therapeutic value.
- Initial management includes physical therapy, nonsteroidal anti-inflammatory drugs, and ultrasound-guided corticosteroid injections; surgery is reserved for refractory cases.
- Arthroscopic release or fractional lengthening provides reliable pain relief and high patient satisfaction with lower complication rates compared to open techniques.

INTRODUCTION

Total hip arthroplasty (THA) is one of the most successful procedures in orthopedic surgery. Since its introduction in the 1960s, it has provided reliable pain relief and functional improvement for patients with advanced degenerative hip disease.[1,2] Over one million THAs are performed worldwide each year, with procedure volume projected to increase further as indications expand and the population ages.[3–7]

Clinical outcomes following THA are excellent, with more than 90% of patients reporting meaningful pain relief and improved function.[8–10] However, as utilization grows, the absolute number of complications continues to rise.[11] Although uncommon, persistent pain after THA is a particularly challenging problem for surgeons to

[a] Department of Orthopedic Surgery and Sports Medicine, Mayo Clinic, 200 First St SW, Rochester, MN, USA; [b] Department of Orthopedic Surgery, Orlando Health Jewett Orthopedic Institute, 60 Columbia St, Orlando, FL, USA
* Corresponding author.
E-mail address: hevesi.mario@mayo.edu

Clin Sports Med 45 (2026) 707–719
https://doi.org/10.1016/j.csm.2026.01.004
sportsmed.theclinics.com
0278-5919/26/

Abbreviations	
AIIS	anterior inferior iliac spine
ASIS	anterior superior iliac spine
IPI	Iliopsoas impingement
NSAID	nonsteroidal anti-inflammatory drug
THA	total hip arthroplasty

address. Common causes include infection, instability, component wear and/or loosening, heterotopic ossification, and soft tissue inflammation (bursitis).[12–17]

Iliopsoas impingement (IPI) is an underrecognized but important etiology to consider in the post-THA patient with pain.[14] Patients typically present with anterior groin pain that worsens with hip flexion and may be associated with snapping.[18–21] The incidence of IPI is reported between 2% and 6% in large series, with a pooled rate near 4%.[22–26] Recognition of this entity is important, as timely diagnosis and targeted treatment can yield excellent outcomes. Treatment options range from conservative measures including physical therapy and diagnostic/therapeutic injections to acetabular component revision in the setting of excessive retroversion, and open or arthroscopic tenotomy.[19,27] This article will discuss pathophysiology, etiology, and surgical options to manage IPI in the post-THA patient.

ANATOMIC CONSIDERATIONS

The iliopsoas tendon is the combined musculotendinous structure of the iliacus and psoas muscles, functioning as the primary hip flexor and a secondary contributor to external rotation of the femur. The psoas muscle contributions consist of the psoas major along with the psoas minor in approximately 60% to 65% of the population.[28,29] These muscles coalesce into a single, bifid, or trifid tendon with approximate frequencies of 28%, 64%, and 8%, respectively (**Fig. 1**).[30] The iliacus originates from the anterior surface of the ilium, while the psoas major arises from the transverse processes and vertebral bodies of L1–L4. The psoas minor, when present, originates from T12–L1 and lies most superficially. These fibers converge to form the iliopsoas tendon, which passes beneath the ilioinguinal ligament, anterior to the acetabular rim, medial

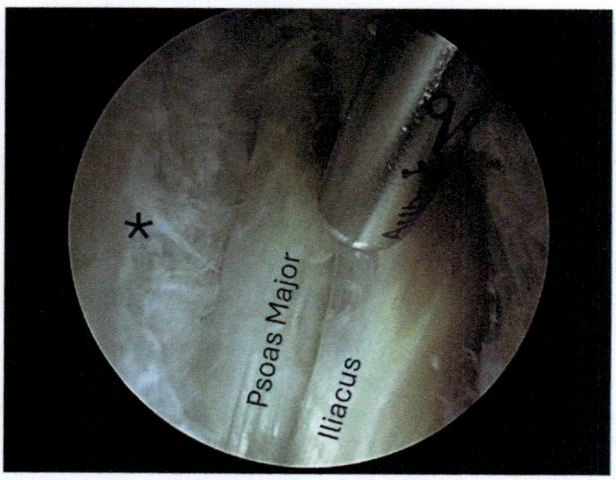

Fig. 1. Arthroscopic visualization of an iliopsoas bifid tendon. Arthroscopic view from the proximal portal with a 70° arthroscope. The bifid iliopsoas tendon is demonstrated, consisting of the psoas major (deep) and iliacus (superficial) portions. The hip capsule is indicated (*asterisk*).

to the anterior superior iliac spine (ASIS), and anterior to the anterior inferior iliac spine (AIIS) and iliocapsularis muscle.[31]

The iliopsoas also defines the lateral border of the femoral triangle. In this region, the femoral nerve lies closest to the tendon, alongside the femoral artery, vein, and branches such as the medial femoral circumflex artery—highlighting the importance of caution with injections or surgical management.[32,33]

As the tendon crosses the anterior acetabular rim (at approximately the 3 o'clock position), its composition is ~40% tendon and ~60% muscle fibers, with tendon fibers situated posterolateral to the surrounding muscle.[34,35] Near the lesser trochanter, this ratio becomes roughly equal. This anatomic course creates 2 potential points of hardware conflict after THA: the acetabular rim and the calcar region prior to insertion on the lesser trochanter. Of note, this calcar region is of increasing importance with the recent popularization of collared, uncemented femoral stems.

Hip flexion is produced by several muscles. The rectus femoris, originating from the AIIS and superior joint capsule, is most active from full extension to ~60° of flexion.[36] The iliopsoas becomes the dominant hip flexor beyond 60° of flexion.[36] This explains classic symptoms of IPI, including difficulty lifting the leg into and out of a car, climbing curbs, or raising the thigh to don socks or pants.[37] Patients may also report pain with coughing or sneezing, weakness from gait compensation, and in some cases, painful snapping of the hip—similar to coxa sultans in the native hip.[20,21,37] Of note, other secondary hip flexors include the sartorius, tensor fascia lata, iliocapsularis, and others.

ETIOLOGY

IPI after THA may result from mechanical irritation between the tendon and prosthetic components. Commonly recognized areas of contact include the anterior acetabular rim and the collar of femoral stems. Other theorized causes include posterolateral displacement of the lesser trochanter, iatrogenic injury, intra-tendon pathology, and anatomic variations.[38]

Acetabular Factors

Early reports of IPI describe patients presenting with anterior groin pain reproduced by resisted hip flexion and straight leg raise.[39–41] Trousdale and colleagues noted symptomatic impingement in patients with anteriorly prominent cups visible on lateral radiographs; symptoms resolved after revision to a recessed (more anteverted) position.[39]

Radiographic thresholds for clinically significant overhang remain debated. True lateral radiographs gauge sagittal prominence, while CT allows for more precise measurements (**Fig. 2**). While initial literature reported axial overhang greater than 12 mm on CT imaging was associated with symptoms, recent evidence identified symptomatic patients with as little as 4 to 6 mm of prominence.[41,42] Ultrasound has also been used, with ≥6 mm prominence proposed as diagnostic.[43] Of note, not all patients with symptomatic iliopsoas tendinitis present with component malposition, as this clinical entity is observed in patients with well-placed components.

As it relates to the acetabular component, several factors may contribute to impingement risk:

- *Cup positioning*: Placement in retroversion, failure to achieve appropriate medialization or component oversizing can increase anterior overhang.[44]
- *Polyethylene Design*: Some polyethylene liner designs lock into the acetabular component in an offset position, whereas while the cup may be recessed under the anterior acetabular rim, the liner may be prominent.

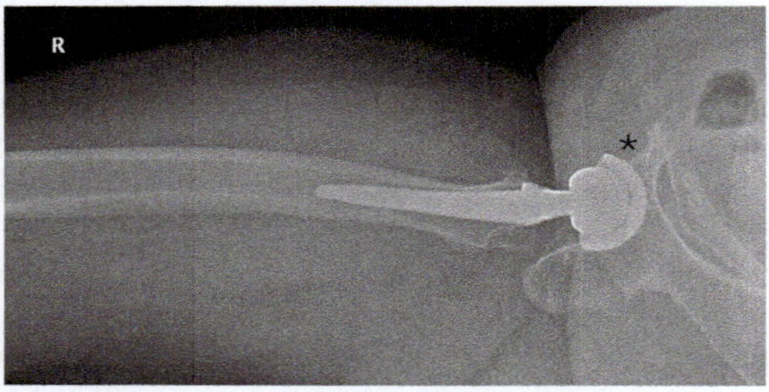

Fig. 2. Acetabular component impingement. Right hip cross-table lateral radiograph demonstrating an acetabular component positioned in excessive retroversion with resultant anterior overhang (*asterisk*).

- *Acetabular Design*: A rough, porous surface intended for bone ingrowth may be abrasive if left exposed.

Thus, acetabular component placement, sizing, and design all play critical roles in the development of IPI. Careful surgical planning and implant selection may minimize risk.

Femoral Factors

In recent years, there has been a trend toward increased adoption of collared femoral stems, particularly in cementless designs. Collared stems have demonstrated lower all-cause revision rates and reduced risk of early periprosthetic fracture by providing calcar support, rotational stability, and assisting with load transfer.[45–47] Despite these advantages, the collar also introduces a potential source of iliopsoas irritation. Medial collar prominence has been associated with IPI, with risk proportional to the degree of overhang.[48] In some systems, collar length scales with stem size (i.e. size specific length), while in others it remains uniform across sizes (i.e. constant length collar). In small femurs, a disproportionately large collar relative to stem size may therefore increase the chance of tendon irritation, though this has not been formally studied (**Fig. 3**A, B).

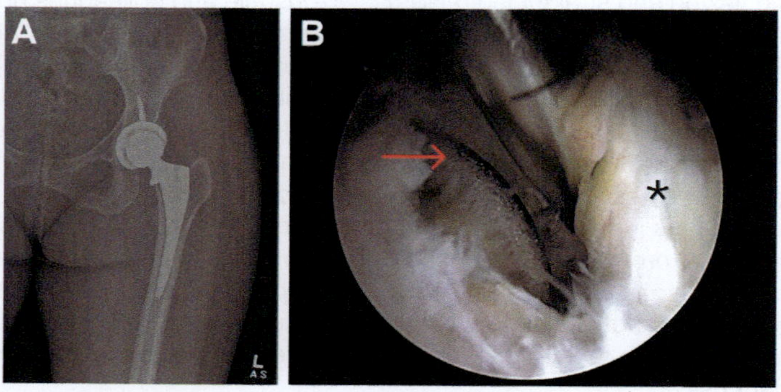

Fig. 3. Femoral collar impingement. (*A*) AP radiograph of a left hip demonstrating a femoral collar protruding beyond the medial femoral calcar. This stem in particular is a size 1, demonstrating the consequence of using an implant with a nonprogressing collar size (i.e. constant length collar) in small femurs. (*B*) Arthroscopic view with a 70° arthroscope identifying a femoral collar (*red arrow*) and its association with the iliopsoas tendon in a right hip (*asterisk*).

Stem alignment can also influence iliopsoas mechanics. Varus placement of straight stems increases hip offset by approximately 1.4 to 1.6 mm for each degree of varus, particularly with a 125° neck angle.[49,50] This altered offset may change tendon trajectory and tension, while also increasing the likelihood of collar prominence medially.

Stem version further contributes to risk. Increased femoral anteversion has been associated with IPI,[48] and cadaveric models demonstrate a direct relationship between anteversion and iliopsoas tension.[51] Greater anteversion displaces the lesser trochanter posterolaterally, increasing torque on the iliopsoas tendon, resulting in a more tortuous course of the tendon to the lesser trochanter, and heightening the risk of impingement against underlying implants. Excessive anteversion may also exacerbate collar overhang in collared designs.

In addition, restoration of offset and leg length must be carefully managed. Both greater offset and leg lengthening have been shown to increase iliopsoas tension, with one large retrospective analysis specifically identifying leg lengthening as an independent risk factor for IPI.[37,51]

Tendon-Specific Pathology

In addition to implant-related factors, intrinsic variation of the iliopsoas tendon may influence the development of tendonitis after THA. The musculotendinous unit arises from the iliacus and psoas muscles, with both psoas major and minor present in most patients. Multifid morphology (bifid or trifid slips) occurs in over 70% of individuals and has been reported at even higher rates among patients requiring surgical treatment for iliopsoas pathology.[28–30,52] Although direct evidence in the arthroplasty population is lacking multifid tendons may predispose to symptomatic snapping and painful tendinitis.

Chronic calcific tendonitis of the iliopsoas, though uncommon, represents another potential source of persistent postoperative pain. It is characterized by groin pain with resisted hip flexion and imaging evidence of focal calcification at the tendon's insertion on the lesser trochanter, in the absence of heterotopic ossification.[53] When symptomatic, management typically involves tendon release with excision of the calcific deposits.[54]

Iatrogenic injury also represents a potential contributor to iliopsoas pathology after THA. Direct trauma to the tendon or muscle belly may occur intraoperatively from retractor placement, particularly during anterior or anterolateral approaches (**Fig. 4**). Excessive or prolonged retraction can lead to stretching or laceration of the iliopsoas, resulting in tendonitis, hematoma, or muscle injury. These changes may produce postoperative groin pain and mimic impingement.[20]

DIAGNOSIS

Clinical Examination

Patients with IPI typically present with anterior groin pain provoked by active—but not passive—hip flexion from a seated position, which is accentuated by resistance. Pain may also be elicited with resisted straight leg raise at 30° to 45° of flexion or at the initiation of walking gait.[18–20] Because hip pain after THA is frequently multifactorial, examination should also screen for infection, loosening, and other sources. Key elements include pain location, systemic signs, weight-bearing tolerance, and provocative maneuvers. In general, CBC, ESR, and CRP remain essential to rule out infection, and if higher suspicion exists, joint aspiration may be helpful. In delayed onset IPI, one may wish to also consider ordering serum metal ion levels to rule metallosis or trunnionosis, if appropriate.

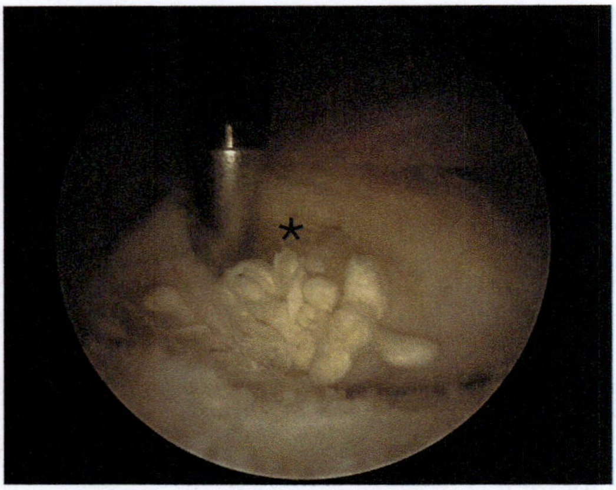

Fig. 4. Iliopsoas tendon trauma. Arthroscopic image during iliopsoas fractional lengthening identifying chronic appearring injury to tendon, consistent with partial tearing (*asterisk*).

Imaging

Initial evaluation should begin with plain radiographs, including anteroposterior (AP) pelvis and crosstable lateral views, to assess for acetabular component orientation and overhang, femoral collar prominence, heterotopic ossification, and signs implant failure (eg, loosening).

CT imaging has been shown to provide more precise characterization of acetabular component orientation, overhang, and screw placement. It can assist with determining femoral version and help better classify the extent of osteophytes or heterotopic ossification as well as rule out component loosening.[27]

MRI may also be helpful in evaluating for iliopsoas tendon pathology. Distortion of its course, hyperintensity on T2 sequences, or associated fluid collections may help with the diagnosis.[37]

Finally, ultrasound offers both diagnostic and therapeutic utility. Dynamic assessment can demonstrate tendon contact with the anterior cup or tendon snapping, while image-guided corticosteroid injection into the tendon sheath can confirm IPI as the pain generator when pain relief follows.[24,38,42]

MANAGEMENT

Initial management is typically nonoperative. A trial of activity modification, nonsteroidal anti-inflammatory drugs (NSAIDs), and structured physical therapy may provide symptomatic relief, especially when coupled with an ultrasound-guided corticosteroid injection.

When symptoms persist despite nonoperative measures, surgical intervention may be indicated. Most authors support allowing sufficient time for postoperative soft tissue irritation to resolve, often which equates to waiting at least 1 year following THA. Surgical strategies include iliopsoas tenotomy or fractional lengthening, as well as revision of the acetabular component in cases of significant malposition. Revision arthroplasty is generally favored in the setting of severely retroverted or oversized cups, loosened implants, or polyethylene wear or failure.[27] In contrast, when acetabular orientation is satisfactory—particularly when anterior prominence is less than 8 mm—arthroscopic iliopsoas tendon lengthening is often the preferred intervention.[27] Of note, recent literature has demonstrated similarly positive outcomes, regardless of degree of anterior acetabular overhang, suggesting that arthroscopic surgical management may be indicated as a first intervention, regardless of the degree of acetabular retroversion, for well-fixed components.[55]

Author's Preferred Technique

The patient is positioned supine on a traction table with the feet secured in padded boots. The operative limb is maintained in approximately 10° of external rotation without distraction. Under fluoroscopic guidance, the level of the lesser trochanter and vastus ridge is marked on the surgical field.

An anterolateral portal is created 2 cm medial to the femoral shaft at the level of the vastus ridge. A 17-gauge spinal needle is advanced from lateral to medial, crossing just medial to the femoral cortex into the iliopsoas bursa. Proper placement is confirmed with an air bursogram, delineating the tendon course (**Fig. 5**A, B). A nitinol wire is inserted, followed by cannula placement under fluoroscopic control. A 70° arthroscope is introduced, and fluid inflow is maintained at low pressure (25–30 mm Hg).

A mid-anterior portal is then established slightly medial and 3 cm distal to the anterolateral portal. After triangulation, a shaver is used to clear bursal tissue and expose the iliopsoas tendon. Fluoroscopy aids in distinguishing the tendon, located posterolateral to the muscle belly, from the adjacent anterior capsule. With the tendon circumferentially defined, a radiofrequency ablator is introduced to perform complete tendon release while preserving underlying muscle. Adequate release is confirmed arthroscopically, with retraction of the tendon ends by 3 to 4 cm (**Fig. 6**A, B).

All instruments are withdrawn, portals are closed in routine fashion, and patients are allowed immediate weight-bearing as tolerated, typically using crutches for 2 to 3 days until pain and gait normalize.

DISCUSSION

The management of IPI after THA has evolved considerably, with both nonoperative and surgical strategies demonstrating success in selected patients. While physical therapy, NSAIDs, and image-guided injections often provide temporary or even durable relief, a subset of patients continue to experience persistent pain requiring surgical intervention. Over the past decade, the literature has increasingly emphasized arthroscopic iliopsoas release as a safe and effective minimally invasive option, though

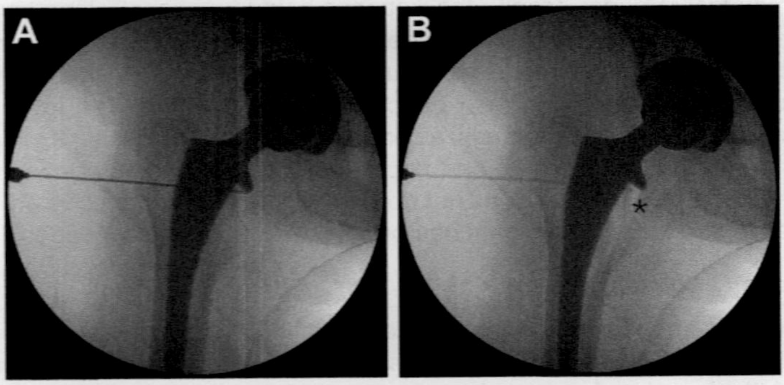

Fig. 5. Iliopsoas air bursogram. (*A*) Fluoroscopic image demonstrating introduction of a 17-gauge spinal needle at the level of the vastus ridge into the area of the iliopsoas bursa with (*B*) subsequent bursogram (*asterisk*) that outlines the iliopsoas tendon sheath.

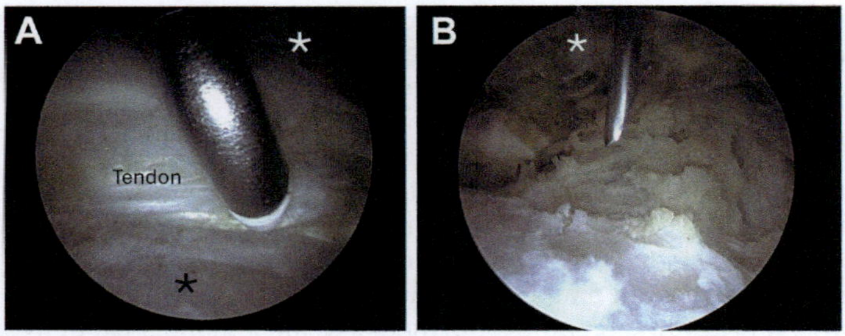

Fig. 6. Arthroscopic tendon release. (*A*) Arthroscopic view of the iliopsoas tendon and its associated muscle belly (*white asterisk*) overlying the hip capsule (*black asterisk*). (*B*) Same view following fractional lengthening where the tendon released leaving the muscular portion intact (*white asterisk*). A spinal 17-gauge spinal needle is then placed to deliver local anesthetic prior to concluding the procedure.

revision of malpositioned components remains necessary in certain cases. Understanding the relative outcomes, risks, and limitations of these treatment strategies is critical to guiding decision-making and counseling patients.

Patient Satisfaction and Outcomes

Both open and arthroscopic approaches to iliopsoas release have demonstrated reliable improvements in pain relief and patient satisfaction. Comparative studies show that while both techniques are effective, arthroscopic tenotomy or lengthening is associated with lower complication and revision rates. As a minimally invasive procedure, arthroscopic release yields favorable results in more than 85% of cases, with groin pain relief reported in over 90% of patients.[20] In addition, significant improvements have been documented in validated outcome measures, including the Harris Hip Score and the Western Ontario and McMaster Universities Osteoarthritis Index.[22,56] These gains, combined with the reduced surgical morbidity of an arthroscopic approach, make it an increasingly preferred option over traditional open techniques.

Patients are routinely counseled that hip flexor weakness may occur following iliopsoas release. Objective testing has, in some series, demonstrated measurable reductions in hip flexion strength after tenotomy. However, most patients report stable or even improved subjective strength. This paradox is likely attributable to the relief of pain, which often limited perceived strength preoperatively; once pain is alleviated, patients may feel stronger despite the iliopsoas being functionally lengthened.[57,58]

Importantly, hip flexion is not solely dependent on the iliopsoas. Other contributors—including the rectus femoris, sartorius, and iliocapsularis—help preserve overall flexion power, mitigating functional deficits after release.[36,59] The level of tendon release may also influence outcomes: a complete release at the lesser trochanter eliminates direct femoral attachment and could theoretically lead to greater weakness. Despite this, current evidence does not consistently demonstrate clinically significant differences in strength or functional outcomes based on release location.

Recurrence and Complications

While outcomes are generally favorable, complications do occur. The most frequently reported issues include persistent groin pain, incomplete symptom relief, or recurrent irritation. Arthroscopic release has been shown to carry lower overall complication and revision rates compared with open surgery, but both approaches can be associated with risks such as hematoma, heterotopic ossification, or over-release leading to hip flexor weakness. Revision surgery may be required in cases of malpositioned acetabular components or when IPI persists despite tendon release or lengthening. Recurrence risk has been reported around 3%.[58] Importantly, instability following tenotomy is rare, but has been described, particularly in the setting of concomitant component malposition or soft tissue deficiency such as that resulting from inside out capsulotomy or capsulectomy at the time of initial arthroscopic visualization of the iliopsoas tendon.[60] Careful patient selection and thorough preoperative counseling remain critical to minimizing these risks.

SUMMARY

IPI is an important and often overlooked cause of groin pain after THA. Careful evaluation—including history, examination, and targeted imaging—is essential to differentiate this pathology from other common etiologies of postoperative hip pain. Most patients respond to conservative measures such as physical therapy, anti-inflammatories, and image-guided corticosteroid injections. For patients who remain symptomatic, surgical treatment may be considered. Arthroscopic iliopsoas release provides a minimally invasive option with high rates of pain relief and patient satisfaction, even in the setting of acetabular component retroversion. Optimal outcomes are achieved through individualized treatment planning.

CLINICS CARE POINTS

- Always exclude infection, loosening, and instability before diagnosing IPI.
- Ultrasound-guided anesthetic and corticosteroid injections are both diagnostic and therapeutic, and can help confirm iliopsoas pathology.
- Arthroscopic iliopsoas fractional lengthening offers approximately 85% patient satisfaction with lower complication rates compared to open release.
- Surgeons should be aware that multiple tendons may exist when performing a release.
- Patients should be counseled preoperatively about the possibility of hip flexor weakness following tenotomy.
- Tendon release at the lesser trochanter may cause greater objective weakness, though functional outcomes are often preserved.

DISCLOSURE

M. Hevesi reports a consulting or advisory relationship with DJO-Enovis, Arthrex, Moximed, Stryker, and Vericel and acknowledges editorial board privileges with *Journal of Cartilage and Joint Preservation*. B.A. Levy reports IP royalties from and paid consultant for Arthrex; stock or stock options with COVR Medical LLC; and editorial or governing board, *Journal of Knee Surgery, Knee Surgery, Sports Traumatology, Arthroscopy, and Orthopedics Today*.

REFERENCES

1. Learmonth ID, Young C, Rorabeck C. The operation of the century: total hip replacement. Lancet 2007;370:1508–19.
2. Lespasio MJ, Sultan AA, Piuzzi NS, et al. Hip osteoarthritis: a primer. Perm J 2018;22:17–084.

3. Singh JA, Yu S, Chen L, et al. Rates of total joint replacement in the United States: future projections to 2020-2040 using the national inpatient sample. J Rheumatol 2019;46:1134–40.
4. Ryan SP, Stambough JB, Huddleston JI 3rd, et al. Highlights of the 2023 American joint replacement registry annual report. Arthroplast Today 2024;26:101325.
5. Ferguson RJ, Palmer AJ, Taylor A, et al. Hip replacement. Lancet 2018;392: 1662–71.
6. Kurtz S, Ong K, Lau E, et al. Projections of primary and revision hip and knee arthroplasty in the United States from 2005 to 2030. J Bone Joint Surg Am 2007;89: 780–5.
7. Shichman I, Roof M, Askew N, et al. Projections and epidemiology of primary hip and knee arthroplasty in medicare patients to 2040-2060. JB JS Open Access 2023;8. https://doi.org/10.2106/JBJS.OA.22.00112.
8. Heath EL, Ackerman IN, Cashman K, et al. Patient-reported outcomes after hip and knee arthroplasty : results from a large national registry. Bone Jt Open 2021;2:422–32.
9. Harris IA, Harris AM, Naylor JM, et al. Discordance between patient and surgeon satisfaction after total joint arthroplasty. J Arthroplast 2013;28:722–7.
10. Anakwe RE, Jenkins PJ, Moran M. Predicting dissatisfaction after total hip arthroplasty: a study of 850 patients. J Arthroplast 2011;26:209–13.
11. Wolf BR, Lu X, Li Y, et al. Adverse outcomes in hip arthroplasty: long-term trends. J Bone Joint Surg Am 2012;94:e103.
12. Bozic KJ, Kurtz SM, Lau E, et al. The epidemiology of revision total hip arthroplasty in the United States. J Bone Joint Surg Am 2009;91:128–33.
13. Legosz P, Otworowski M, Sibilska A, et al. Heterotopic ossification: a challenging complication of total hip arthroplasty: risk factors, diagnosis, prophylaxis, and treatment. BioMed Res Int 2019;3860142. https://doi.org/10.1155/2019/3860142.
14. Hevesi M, Simon KN, Lachman N, et al. Iliopsoas tendonitis and impingement after total hip arthroplasty. J Am Acad Orthop Surg 2025. https://doi.org/10.5435/JAAOS-D-25-00476.
15. Nam D, Nunley RM, Sauber TJ, et al. Incidence and location of pain in young, active patients following hip arthroplasty. J Arthroplast 2015;30:1971–5.
16. Li T, Li Y, Wang W. Association between cup orientation and low back pain after total hip arthroplasty in patients with osteonecrosis of the femoral head. BMC Musculoskelet Disord 2024;25:10.
17. Axelrod DE, Ekhtiari S, Winemaker MJ, et al. Management of greater trochanteric pain syndrome after total hip arthroplasty: practice patterns and surgeon attitudes. J Am Acad Orthop Surg Glob Res Rev 2023;7. https://doi.org/10.5435/JAAOSGlobal-D-23-00085.
18. Bricteux S, Beguin L, Fessy MH. [Iliopsoas impingement in 12 patients with a total hip arthroplasty]. Rev Chir Orthop Reparatrice Appar Mot 2001;87:820–5.
19. O'Sullivan M, Tai CC, Richards S, et al. Iliopsoas tendonitis a complication after total hip arthroplasty. J Arthroplast 2007;22:166–70.
20. May O. Arthroscopic techniques for treating ilio-psoas tendinopathy after hip arthroplasty. Orthop Traumatol Surg Res 2019;105:S177–85.
21. Bardakos NV. Hip impingement: beyond femoroacetabular. J Hip Preserv Surg 2015;2:206–23.
22. Zimmerer A, Hauschild M, Nietschke R, et al. Results after arthroscopic treatment of iliopsoas impingement after total hip arthroplasty. Arch Orthop Trauma Surg 2022;142:189–95.

23. Bartelt RB, Yuan BJ, Trousdale RT, et al. The prevalence of groin pain after metal-on-metal total hip arthroplasty and total hip resurfacing. Clin Orthop Relat Res 2010;468:2346–56.
24. Ala Eddine T, Remy F, Chantelot C, et al. [Anterior iliopsoas impingement after total hip arthroplasty: diagnosis and conservative treatment in 9 cases]. Rev Chir Orthop Reparatrice Appar Mot 2001;87:815–9.
25. Verhaegen JCF, Vandeputte FJ, Van den Broecke R, et al. Risk factors for iliopsoas tendinopathy after anterior approach total hip arthroplasty. J Arthroplast 2023;38:511–8.
26. Buller LT, Menken LG, Hawkins EJ, et al. Iliopsoas impingement after direct anterior approach total hip arthroplasty: epidemiology, risk factors, and treatment options. J Arthroplast 2021;36:1772–8.
27. Chalmers BP, Sculco PK, Sierra RJ, et al. Iliopsoas impingement after primary total hip arthroplasty: operative and nonoperative treatment outcomes. J Bone Joint Surg Am 2017;99:557–64.
28. Neumann DA, Garceau LR. A proposed novel function of the psoas minor revealed through cadaver dissection. Clin Anat 2015;28:243–52.
29. Anderson CN. Iliopsoas: pathology, diagnosis, and treatment. Clin Sports Med 2016;35:419–33.
30. Philippon MJ, Devitt BM, Campbell KJ, et al. Anatomic variance of the iliopsoas tendon. Am J Sports Med 2014;42:807–11.
31. Lin B, Bartlett J, Lloyd TD, et al. Multiple iliopsoas tendons: a cadaveric study and treatment implications for internal snapping hip syndrome. Arch Orthop Trauma Surg 2022;142:1147–54.
32. Lonchena TK, McFadden K, Orebaugh SL. Correlation of ultrasound appearance, gross anatomy, and histology of the femoral nerve at the femoral triangle. Surg Radiol Anat 2016;38:115–22.
33. Orebaugh SL. The femoral nerve and its relationship to the lateral circumflex femoral artery. Anesth Analg 2006;102:1859–62.
34. Blomberg JR, Zellner BS, Keene JS. Cross-sectional analysis of iliopsoas muscle-tendon units at the sites of arthroscopic tenotomies: an anatomic study. Am J Sports Med 2011;39(Suppl):58S–63S.
35. Alpert JM, Kozanek M, Li G, et al. Cross-sectional analysis of the iliopsoas tendon and its relationship to the acetabular labrum: an anatomic study. Am J Sports Med 2009;37:1594–8.
36. Kumazaki T, Takahashi T, Nakano T, et al. Action and contribution of the iliopsoas and rectus femoris as hip flexor agonists examined with anatomical analysis. Juntendo Iji Zasshi 2022;68:352–62.
37. Park CW, Yoo I, Cho K, et al. Incidence and risk factors of iliopsoas tendinopathy after total hip arthroplasty: a radiographic analysis of 1,602 hips. J Arthroplast 2023;38:1621–7.
38. Lequesne M, Dang N, Montagne P, et al. [Conflict between psoas and total hip prosthesis]. Rev Rhum Mal Osteoartic 1991;58:559–64.
39. Trousdale RT, Cabanela ME, Berry DJ. Anterior iliopsoas impingement after total hip arthroplasty. J Arthroplast 1995;10:546–9.
40. Postel M, Painful prosthesis I. Possible causes]. Rev Chir Orthop Reparatrice Appar Mot 1975;61(Suppl 2):57–61.
41. Cyteval C, Sarrabère MP, Cottin A, et al. Iliopsoas impingement on the acetabular component: radiologic and computed tomography findings of a rare hip prosthesis complication in eight cases. J Comput Assist Tomogr 2003;27:183–8.

42. Ueno T, Kabata T, Kajino Y, et al. Risk factors and cup protrusion thresholds for symptomatic iliopsoas impingement after total hip arthroplasty: a retrospective case-control study. J Arthroplast 2018;33:3288–96.e1.
43. Guillin R, Bertaud V, Garetier M, et al. Ultrasound in total hip replacement: value of anterior acetabular cup visibility and contact with the iliopsoas tendon. J Ultrasound Med 2018;37:1439–46.
44. Abbas AA, Kim YJ, Song EK, et al. Oversized acetabular socket causing groin pain after total hip arthroplasty. J Arthroplast 2009;24:1144–8.e5.
45. Lamb JN, Baetz J, Messer-Hannemann P, et al. A calcar collar is protective against early periprosthetic femoral fracture around cementless femoral components in primary total hip arthroplasty: a registry study with biomechanical validation. Bone Joint J 2019;101-b:779–86.
46. Rele S, O'Bryan E, Holder C, et al. Collared cementless femoral components reduce the revision rates in primary total hip arthroplasty using the direct anterior approach: an Australian orthopaedic Association national joint replacement registry study. J Arthroplast 2024;39:340–6.e2.
47. Rodriguez S, Puri S, Bido J, et al. How much protection does a collar provide? Assessing risk of early periprosthetic femur fractures following total hip arthroplasty in elderly patients. J Arthroplast 2024;39:997–1000.e1.
48. Qiu J, Ke X, Chen S, et al. Risk factors for iliopsoas impingement after total hip arthroplasty using a collared femoral prosthesis. J Orthop Surg Res 2020;15:267.
49. Luger M, Stiftinger J, Allerstorfer J, et al. High varus stem alignment in short-stem total hip arthroplasty: a risk for reconstruction of femoro-acetabular offset, leg length discrepancy and stem undersizing? Arch Orthop Trauma Surg 2022;142:2935–44.
50. Maurer-Ertl W, Friesenbichler J, Pfann M, et al. Restoration of hip geometry after total hip arthroplasty: retrospective comparison of two short stems and one straight stem. BMC Musculoskelet Disord 2022;23:1035.
51. Tamaki Y, Goto T, Iwase J, et al. Relationship between iliopsoas muscle surface pressure and implant alignment after total hip arthroplasty: a cadaveric study. Sci Rep 2023;13:3492.
52. Hwang A, Martinez M, Cora Jones CM, et al. Multifid iliopsoas tendons are more common in patients with painful snapping iliopsoas tendons. Arthrosc Sports Med Rehabil 2023;5:100780.
53. Henry S, Small T, Cottle D. Unusual presentation of calcific tendinitis of the iliopsoas tendon in a 28-year-old female. ANZ J Surg 2019;89:E398–9.
54. Park SM, Baek JH, Ko YB, et al. Management of acute calcific tendinitis around the hip joint. Am J Sports Med 2014;42:2659–65.
55. Simon KN, Jurgensmeier K, Vogel M, et al. Arthroscopic fractional lengthening after total hip arthroplasty results in improved patient-reported outcomes and low rates of revision total hip arthroplasty. Arthrosc Sports Med Rehabil 2024;6:100930.
56. Shapira J, Chen SL, Wojnowski NM, et al. Outcomes of nonoperative management, iliopsoas tenotomy, and revision arthroplasty for iliopsoas impingement after total hip arthroplasty: a systematic review. J Arthroplast 2019;34:2184–91.
57. Portet A, Repellin M, Lambrey PJ, et al. Assessment of function and muscle strength after endoscopic iliopsoas tenotomy to treat iliopsoas impingement after total hip arthroplasty. Int Orthop 2024;48:2375–82.
58. Finsterwald M, Mancino F, Waters G, et al. Endoscopic tendon release for iliopsoas impingement after total hip arthroplasty-excellent clinical outcomes and low failure rates at short-term Follow-Up. Arthroscopy 2024;40:790–8.

59. Lawrenson P, Hodges P, Crossley K, et al. The effect of altered stride length on iliocapsularis and pericapsular muscles of the anterior hip: an electromyography investigation during asymptomatic gait. Gait Posture 2019;71:26–31.
60. Yoon SJ, Ko JH, Matsuda DK. Anterior dislocation of THA after iliopsoas tenotomy in spinopelvic imbalance: a rare case report. BMC Musculoskelet Disord 2020; 21:723.

Deep Gluteal Space Anatomy, Pathology, Clinical Presentation, and Management

Joshua D. Harris, MD[a,b,*]

KEYWORDS

- Deep gluteal space • Ischiofemoral • Hamstring • Sciatic
- Posterior femoral cutaneous • Piriformis • Sacroiliac

KEY POINTS

- There are multiple different osseous and soft tissue causes of posterior hip pain, including the deep gluteal space, lumbosacral spine, hip joint, and intrapelvis, either in isolation or combination.
- A systematic approach to the clinical presentation and imaging requires exhaustive patience, as most patients have had several years of significant symptoms, seen multiple physicians, been given multiple differing diagnoses, and attempted multiple independent treatments without success.
- Selective injections are beneficial when positive—ischiofemoral space, quadratus femoris, obturator internus, piriformis, sacroiliac joint, lumbosacral spine, hip joint.
- Advanced imaging routinely includes MRI (including neurography) of the pelvis and lumbosacral spine and computed tomography of the pelvis (including version analysis and 3 dimensional reconstruction) with the feet positioned as in the mid-stance phase of gait.
- In the event of inability to satisfactorily improve symptoms with nonsurgical treatment, surgical treatment choices include a variety of endoscopic and open approaches, either in isolation or combination, either simultaneously or staged.

INTRODUCTION

The deep gluteal space is a highly complex anatomic region bounded by both osseous and soft tissue structures. Contained within the space itself are dozens of musculotendinous, neurovascular, and osseous entities that may account for pain directly from that region. The relatively high frequency of variant anatomy makes the space even more challenging to understand and manage. Compounded with this intricate posterior hip anatomy is the fact that many individuals with pain perceived here may simply

[a] Department of Orthopaedics & Sports Medicine, 6445 Main Street, Houston, TX 77030, USA; [b] Department of Orthopaedic Surgery, Weill Cornell Medical College, New York, NY 10065, USA
* Department of Orthopaedics & Sports Medicine, 6445 Main Street, Houston, TX 77030.
E-mail address: joshuaharrismd@gmail.com

Clin Sports Med 45 (2026) 721–734
https://doi.org/10.1016/j.csm.2026.01.005 sportsmed.theclinics.com
0278-5919/26/

Abbreviations

AP	anteroposterior
CT	computed tomography
IFI	ischiofemoral impingement
FAI	femoroacetabular impingement
SI	sacroiliac

be perceiving it there because of referred pain patterns from the lumbar spine, lumbosacral plexus, hip joint, or within the pelvis. The deep gluteal space was first reported in the literature in 1999.[1] Analogous to "sports hernia" (also known as athletic pubalgia, inguinal disruption, core muscle injury, among several others), deep gluteal syndrome has been labeled with several other vague, generic, imprecise, and unintentionally misleading other names including piriformis syndrome, sciatica, pseudosciatica, sciatic neuropathy, posterior hip pain, buttock pain, pelvic outlet syndrome, wallet syndrome, gemelli-obturator syndrome, ischiofemoral impingement (IFI) syndrome, proximal hamstring syndrome, among others. The heterogeneity in nomenclature is likely attributable to the difficult diagnosis. Despite two and a half decades of clinical experience and research, consistent and accurate anatomic diagnosis with resultant reliable and successful treatment remains elusive.

ANATOMY

The deep gluteal space bears its name secondary to its posterior border, or roof from a prone position, the gluteus maximus. The anterior border is the posterior hip joint, posterior column of the pelvis, and the proximal femur. The lateral border is the gluteus maximus insertion on the posterior femur. The medial border is the sacrotuberous ligament, the medial margin of the proximal hamstring origin, and the adductor magnus origin. The superior border is the piriformis muscle entry into the greater sciatic foramen. The inferior border is the proximal hamstring origin on the ischial tuberosity. Within the space include several muscles (piriformis, superior and inferior gemelli, obturator internus and externus, quadratus femoris, proximal hamstring, and adductor magnus), nerves (sciatic, superior and inferior gluteal, posterior femoral cutaneous, and pudendal), vessels (perineural/sciatic/posterior femoral cutaneous vasculature, and perforator branches), and bursa (ischial).

Neural structures of the deep gluteal space exiting the greater sciatic foramen are often cited as sources of pain in deep gluteal syndrome. Nerves exiting below piriformis include the sciatic nerve, posterior femoral cutaneous nerve, pudendal nerve, inferior gluteal nerve, nerve to obturator internus, and nerve to quadratus femoris. The only nerve to exit above the piriformis is the superior gluteal nerve. In the context of posterior hip pain treatment, the surgeon must be cognizant of normal anatomy, anatomic variations, and abnormal fibrous/fibrovascular/vascular bands that mimic or parallel normal neurovascular structures.

The most common pertinent variation in the deep gluteal space is variant sciatic nerve anatomy. The normal sciatic nerve includes the terminal branches of the ventral rami of L4 through S3. There are 2 divisions within the nerve—tibial (medial) and common peroneal (lateral). There are 6 known different sciatic nerve variants, 4 of which were observed in the original classification proposed by Beaton & Anson, varying based on their path relative to the piriformis muscle[2]—(1) undivided nerve passing completely below piriformis (83.1%); (2) divided nerve passing through (common peroneal portion) and below (tibial portion) piriformis (13.7%); (3) divided nerve passing above (common peroneal portion) and below (tibial portion) piriformis (1.3%); (4)

undivided nerve passing completely through piriformis (0.5%); (5) divided nerve passing above (common peroneal portion) and through (tibial portion) piriformis (0.08%); and (6) undivided nerve passing completely above piriformis (0.08%).[3] Nearly two-thirds (63.6%) of specimens had bilateral sciatic nerve/piriformis anomalous anatomy.[3] Given that 16.9% (n = 1024) of 6062 dissected cadaveric *limbs* had a variant in sciatic nerve/piriformis anatomy and 63.6% of those variants were bilateral, the prevalence of at least one anomaly in an individual specimen was 23.1%.[3]

There are 3 types of bands that may constrict excursion of the sciatic nerve in the deep gluteal space: fibrovascular bands, purely fibrous bands without macroscopically visible vessels, and purely vascular bands without macroscopically visible fibrous tissue.[4] The location of these bands may be classified using their location: proximal (just exiting greater sciatic foramen), middle (from piriformis to obturator internus), and distal (at level of quadratus femoris and proximal hamstring).[4] They can be further subdivided as medial, lateral, or both medial and lateral to the sciatic nerve.[4] Pertinent to the mechanism of nerve involvement, there are 3 types of bands: type 1 (compressive, bridge-type; 1a compresses from anterior to posterior; 1b compresses from posterior to anterior); type 2 (adhesive, horse-type; single binding location to the nerve from either lateral at the greater trochanter [2a; more common] or medial at the sacrotuberous ligament [2b; less common]); and type 3 (random, erratic, variable attachment points).[4] Especially pertinent to understanding the difference between normal anatomy and abnormal truly pathologic symptom-causing fibrous/fibrovascular/vascular bands are the first branches off the sciatic nerve to innervate the long head biceps femoris (mean 6.9 cm), semitendinosus (mean 7.1 cm), semimembranosus (mean 13.1 cm), adductor magnus (mean 13.1 cm), and short head biceps femoris (mean 14 cm).[5,6] In addition to bands that restrict motion of the sciatic nerve, fibrous/fibrovascular/vascular bands may also constrict excursion of the posterior femoral cutaneous nerve (**Fig. 1**).

CLINICAL PRESENTATION

Patients with posterior hip pain present a diagnostic challenge due to a variety of symptoms and signs that may emanate from a combination of different hip layers

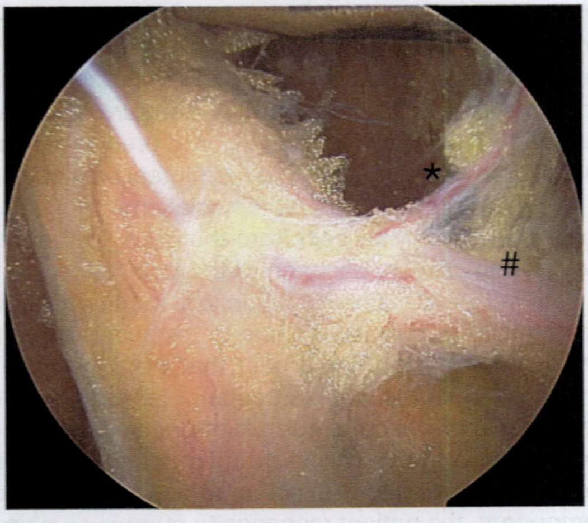

Fig. 1. Right deep gluteal space endoscopy, showing vascular band (*asterisk*) and fibrovascular band (#) both attached to the underlying posterior femoral cutaneous nerve.

and also from several extra-articular sources including the lumbosacral spine, pelvis, peritrochanteric space, and deep gluteal space. Importantly, there is not one focal location that is always symptomatic in patients with deep gluteal space pain. The pain location varies frequently secondary to the underlying causative pathology. Frequently, buttock pain is a common chief complaint. The clinician must iteratively inquire the exact precise location, as many patients will say "glute pain" or "gluteal pain," rather than buttock pain. This may be misinterpreted as lateral/peritrochanteric hip from gluteus medius/minimus and/or greater trochanteric bursa. Pain duration is typically quite long, longer than that of femoroacetabular impingement (FAI) syndrome, acetabular dysplasia, or arthritis. Multiple visits to physicians in different specialties are common—primary care physician, orthopedic surgeon (general, sports medicine, adult reconstruction, hip preservation, spine), neurologic surgeon (spine), general surgeon, obstetrician/gynecologist, urologist, pain management/anesthesiologist, and psychiatrist/mental health/behavioral specialist. Many patients will have been given a variety of plausible and implausible diagnoses in and around the deep gluteal space. Most patients will have attempted several treatments, both nonsurgical and surgical, some even without being given a diagnosis. From a surgical perspective, unfortunately, lumbar spine and sacroiliac (SI) surgeries have often been performed due to buttock pain and "abnormal" lumbosacral spine imaging findings. Analogous to the hip joint, there is a high prevalence of incidental abnormal imaging findings in asymptomatic individuals' lumbar spines. Thus, it is not unreasonable to presume that, without accurate diagnosis, persistent pain leads to desperate patients and attempts at surgical treatment based on erroneous lumbosacral spine imaging findings. These surgeries include lumbosacral fusion and SI "fusion." Unfortunately, both of these typically not only permit continuing pain, but also usually worsen the pain secondary to worsening IFI.

Deep gluteal syndrome has been previously defined as nondiscogenic sciatic nerve disorder with entrapment in the deep gluteal space.[7] Unfortunately, this definition does little to identify or characterize the nociceptive source of the constellation of symptoms defining the syndrome. Many patients have been generically diagnosed with piriformis syndrome. The concept of piriformis syndrome has been reported in the literature since 1928.[8] It was first reported as "pyriformis syndrome" in 1947.[9] One can infer that piriformis syndrome's source of nociception is the piriformis muscle itself. Thus, piriformis syndrome can cause posterior hip pain. However, not all posterior hip pain is piriformis syndrome. Unfortunately, many clinicians generically call all posterior hip pain "piriformis syndrome." Due to this imprecision, in 1999,[1] the phrase "deep gluteal syndrome" was introduced in the literature in order to improve diagnostic clarity–albeit better, it still fails to properly and precisely give a clear diagnosis. Importantly, the pain source in patients with deep gluteal pain can come from a variety of nerve, muscle, or other sources, not just the sciatic nerve.

Optimal diagnosis in patients with pain from the deep gluteal space begins with a thorough history of present illness. Location of the pain helps, but does not typically yield the answer. Pain frequently is neuropathic (eg, burning, stinging, tingling, prickling, electric shocks, numbness, radiating) due to the sciatic and/or posterior femoral cutaneous pudendal nerve(s).[10,11] Nerve pain that goes below the knee is usually sciatic in etiology, while above the knee is posterior femoral cutaneous. A significant positive response (ie, relief of the chief complaint pain location) to a local anesthetic injection in the deep gluteal space is often confirmatory for the diagnostic location of symptoms. As opposed to a hip joint injection, which does not usually have a numbness symptom component, the patient response to numbing a pain source around the sciatic or posterior femoral cutaneous nerve(s) may be difficult to interpret. If the chief complaint significantly improves (>50%–75%) when you directly inquire about the precise pain location, then that location can be assumed to causatively participating in the symptoms. This does not mean that the nerve itself is the etiology of the pain, just that the pathoanatomic location is. This location may be the symptom source due to osseous (eg, IFI from the lesser and/or greater trochanters, femoral neck) or soft tissue (eg, fibrovascular bands) reasons.

Gait assessment is critically important to making an accurate diagnosis. An antalgic gait, despite its frequency observed in hip joint pathology, is infrequently seen in deep gluteal pain. A Trendelenburg gait is very common—in fact, it may be the most common. Peritrochanteric pain (eg, gluteus medius tear, greater trochanteric bursitis, and abductor fatigue from dysplasia) is the inciting pain source, with weak abduction permitting contralateral pelvic tilt and narrowing of the ischiofemoral space, resulting in deep gluteal pain.[12] A shortened stride is often observed due to a loss of hip extension secondary to lesser trochanteric IFI.[13] Since the pelvis can be considered the bottom vertebral level,[14] prior lumbar spine fusion locks typically mobile vertebral segments, preventing the ischium from clearing out of the way of the femur with the extension phase of gait, resulting in a shortened stride and lesser trochanteric IFI (an excellent example of hip-spine syndrome[15]). In-toeing gait is a very specific indicator for excessive femoral anteversion, which results in the posterior intertrochanteric line being in closer proximity to the ischium with resultant IFI.[16] While not all patients with elevated femoral version in-toe, nearly all in-toeing individuals have excessive femoral anteversion.[17] A lack of ability to sit with the symptomatic leg crossed over the other (ipsilateral foot/ankle on contralateral knee) is commonly due to greater trochanteric IFI.[18]

Low back pain is one of the most common presenting complaints, often due to the mechanical stress transmission from the femur colliding into the ischium/pelvis and being sent across the SI joint into the lumbar spine.[19] Prior lumbar spine fusion locks typically mobile vertebral segments, preventing the ischium from clearing out of the way of the femur with the extension phase of gait, resulting in a shortened stride and lesser trochanteric IFI. Sacroiliac "fusion" is often a misnomer, considering no actual fusion mass results from fixation across the synovial joint with a variety of implants without removal of the articulating cartilage surfaces. In fact, given the rapid increase in the incidence of this procedure, a concurrent increase in L5 and S1 nerve root complications has also been observed (**Fig. 2**A–C). Total hip replacement with reduced femoral offset narrows the ischiofemoral space and leads to deep gluteal space pain from IFI. Even with an apparently seemingly normal ischiofemoral space on the AP (anteroposterior) pelvis plain radiograph, the ischiofemoral space can be quite narrow (**Fig. 3**A, B). Unfortunately, many patients undergo total hip arthroplasty

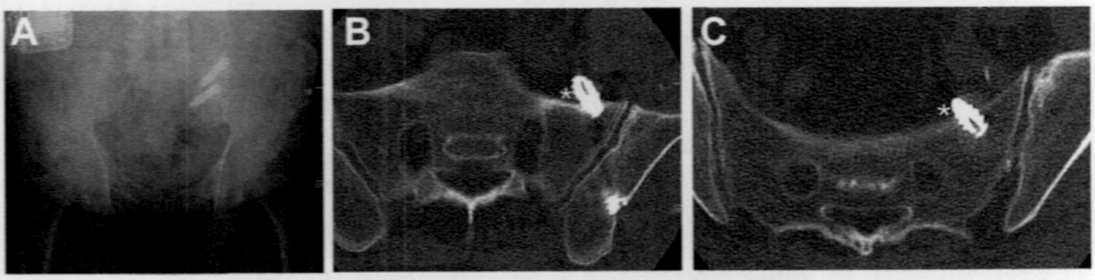

Fig. 2. (*A*) Anteroposterior pelvis plain radiograph demonstrating 2 sacroiliac fixation devices in the left sacroiliac joint of a 52 year old man; (*B*) same patient as A, with the screw contacting the left L5 nerve root (*); (*C*) same patient as A, with the screw contacting the left S1 nerve root (*).

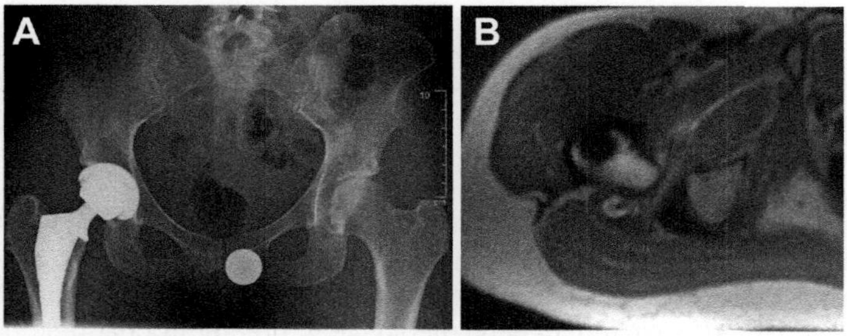

Fig. 3. (*A*) Anteroposterior pelvis plain radiograph demonstrating right total hip arthroplasty in a 40 year old woman. (*B*) Axial T1 magnetic resonance image of same patient in A, with severe ischiofemoral narrowing, despite the plain radiograph showing an apparently open ischiofemoral space. Importantly, foot position during the pelvis radiograph was forced internal rotation and during the MRI was neutral. The patient ambulated with a neutral foot progression angle (~0° at mid-stance phase of gait).

for an inaccurate preoperative diagnosis of hip joint pain from arthritis, when in actuality it was deep gluteal space pain as the symptom source. Not only does this fail to relieve symptoms, but if offset is narrowed further, it only exacerbates symptom severity. Sitting intolerance is very common, usually due to burning pain over the gluteal crease due to the posterior femoral cutaneous nerve (transverse branch > vertical branch) role in deep gluteal space. Patients with low sitting tolerance often stand throughout clinical encounters or sit on a variety of pillows, cushions, or "donuts." Hamstring symptoms ("sit bone" pain) are not infrequent, especially high-grade partial thickness proximal hamstring tears and tendinopathy due to repetitive friction with ambulation from IFI in the deep gluteal space (**Fig. 4**). Pain on the tuberosity is frequently from the proximal hamstring tendon, lateral to the tuberosity attributed to the deep gluteal and ischiofemoral spaces, and medial to the tuberosity attributed to the pudendal nerve.

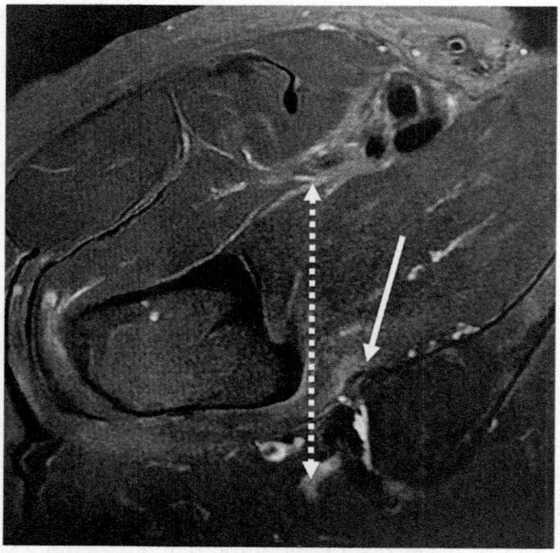

Fig. 4. Axial T2 magnetic resonance image of 41 year old female runner demonstrating an anterior semimembranosus tear (*arrow* with *straight line*) secondary to ischiofemoral impingement mechanism (*arrow* with *dotted line*).

IMAGING

Plain radiographs are the initial modality used to visualize the structure of the hip, pelvis, and lumbosacral spine. Standing AP pelvis, false profile, and Dunn 45° lateral are the hip/pelvis series obtained. Lumbosacral imaging includes AP, lateral, and oblique views. Pertinent imaging findings in the deep gluteal space include sclerosis on the lateral ischial tuberosity (reactive process from IFI), valgus neck shaft angle (either true hip valgus or excessive femoral anteversion), and narrowed ischiofemoral space (either false profile or AP pelvis view). In individuals with prior surgery, pertinent findings include prior spine/SI instrumentation, prior hip fracture fixation (eg, intramedullary nail, plate/screw construct), and prior total hip arthroplasty.

MRI should include, at a minimum, dedicated pelvis and lumbosacral spine series. Pertinent findings in the pelvis should be based on both fluid-sensitive and fat-sensitive techniques. On axial series, narrowing of the ischiofemoral space is characteristic of IFI (both lesser and greater trochanters). Edema in and atrophy of the quadratus femoris are also IFI (lesser trochanter) findings. Proximal hamstring tendon pathology (tendinosis, partial and full-thickness tears) is often observed. As an incipient cause of deep gluteal space pain, abductor tendon pathology may also be seen on pelvis MRI. One may gain insight into the length of time necessary to generate the posterior pain if caused by the lateral hip based on the degree of atrophy and/or fibrofatty infiltration of the abductor muscles (modified Goutallier-Fuchs classification system).[20] Pelvis imaging may also visualize structures outside of the deep gluteal space that can cause pain there—common causes of pain here with or without true sciatica include endometriosis, ovarian cyst, tumor, infection, and SI joint. Although routine pelvis MRI series can visualize the course of the sciatic and posterior femoral cutaneous nerves, MRI neurography series can better visualize the posterior nerves, including the lumbosacral plexus, and, with greater sensitivity, detect pathology in and around the nerves themselves. One of the most important aspects of MRI (and computed tomography [CT]) axial imaging is assurance of the feet positioned to best represent the mid-stance phase of gait (if patient in-toes, then foot position in scanner should be in-toed to that exact amount; if patient out-toes, then foot position should be represented in that exact amount of out-toeing foot progression angle). Simply tying the feet together with toes straight up and down does not accurately portray ischiofemoral space anatomy. Since most deep gluteal space disorders, especially IFI, are dynamic, advanced imaging should attempt to best represent this with proper foot positioning. Positional MRI sequences are available in some institutions to better portray IFI (**Fig. 5**)—internal and external limb rotation, and FABER (flexion, abduction, and external rotation).

CT should include whole pelvis and distal femur series at a minimum. This permits measurement of femoral and acetabular version, with 3 dimensional reconstructions. Collision detection software may take advantage of this osseous imaging modality, either with proprietary software or even simple and cost-effective commercially available 3D printers. Just like MRI, foot position in the scanner should be the same as the mid-stance phase of gait. Pelvis CT may also give valuable information regarding pelvic incidence, pelvic tilt, and sacral slope using the lateral scout view; and leg length evaluation using the AP scout view. If prior SI fixation was performed, it can precisely visualize hardware and proximity to lumbosacral nerve roots, especially L5. CT also has a valuable role in deep gluteal space injections–between lesser trochanter and ischium for IFI (lesser trochanter), at the obturator internus groove just above the proximal hamstring origin for IFI (greater trochanter), at the piriformis for suspected piriformis syndrome (local anesthetic, corticosteroid, Botox [onabotulinumtoxinA]), and SI

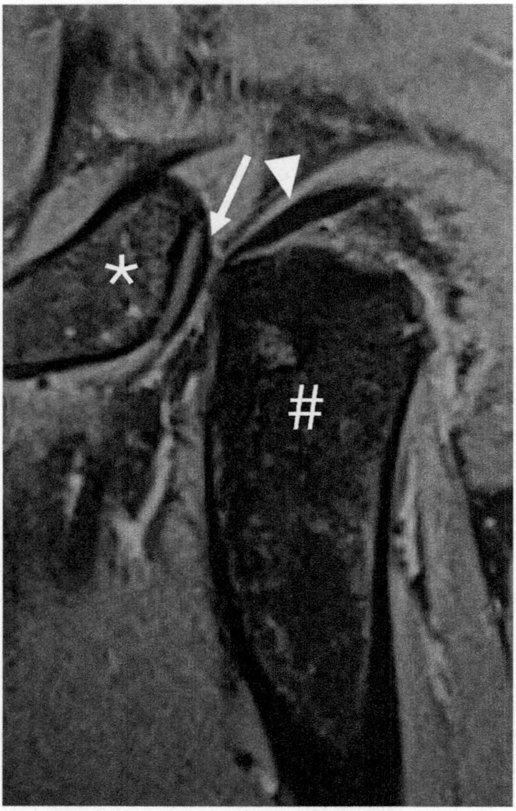

Fig. 5. FABER (flexion, abduction, external rotation) positional magnetic resonance image in 30 year old female right hip demonstrating greater trochanter (#)—ischium (*asterisk*) ischiofemoral impingement; arrowhead indicates gluteus medius tendon; arrow indicates proximal hamstring tendon.

joint (usually lower 1/3 of joint where an actual space in the synovial joint may permit 0.5–2.0 mL of fluid injection).

TREATMENT

The mainstay of nonsurgical treatment is education-driven personalized physical therapy with a home exercise program and activity modification. A clear and concise understanding of etiology is necessary to have the best chance of nonsurgical symptom improvement. If abductor pathology is the underlying incipient cause, with a resultant Trendelenburg gait, the solution is abduction strength while ambulating to prevent dynamic IFI. This frequently necessitates pain improvement in both the posterior and lateral hip. This usually means that the majority of physical therapy is strengthening with minimal/no stretching. Importantly, strength exercises for abduction must avoid intentionally (or unintentionally) causing IFI (greater trochanter)—common provocative ones include the clamshell, fire hydrant, and side-lying leg lift. If IFI from the lesser trochanter is the source of deep gluteal pain, then gait optimization typically includes encouraged shorter abducted strides with the limb internally rotated. If IFI from the greater trochanter is the pain source, avoidance of **Fig. 4** seated positions and "turn out" FABER sitting is recommended. If the hip joint and/or lumbosacral spine are concurrently involved, then they too must be treated.

Medical treatment includes oral nonopioid, nonsteroidal anti-inflammatory medications and selective injections (eg, ischiofemoral space, hip joint, lumbosacral spine, peritrochanteric/lateral hip, and SI joint). With neuropathic pain, medications like gabapentin (Neurontin) and pregabalin (Lyrica) may be used. Finding a balance between the benefit of pain relief and the risks of side effects with nerve medications is critical. The most common significant side effects include sedation/tiredness/fatigue/somnolence, lightheadedness/dizziness/imbalance, and weight gain/swelling/peripheral edema. Common pertinent side effects of nonsteroidal anti-inflammatory use include gastrointestinal (gastritis, ulcer [gastric, duodenal], bleeding), both renal and hepatic, and cardiovascular.

For surgical treatment, endoscopic or open management of the deep gluteal space may be performed in isolation or combination with other hip procedures either simultaneously or in staged fashion. If the hip joint is the pain source (eg, arthritis, dysplasia, FAI) and abductor dysfunction occurs secondary to the joint, then joint treatment(s) is/are warranted, including hip arthroscopy, total hip arthroplasty, and periacetabular osteotomy. If total hip replacement has already been performed and may be causative in posterior symptoms, then revision may be indicated–acetabular cup revision, offset liner, femoral stem revision (increased offset, conical stem derotation if excessively anteverted). The balance of intraoperative complication risk (especially femoral stem revision) must be carefully considered. If femoral stem revision is performed, careful templating, 3 dimensional modeling, and intraoperative robotic navigation can reduce risk of significant leg length discrepancy. Also, if abductor tendon pathology also present, then increased femoral offset may exacerbate the lateral hip. If an abductor tendon tear is present and symptomatic, it should be concomitantly surgically treated with anatomic repair. If excessive femoral anteversion is an underlying structural problem, then derotational osteotomy may be indicated. Similarly, valgus neck-shaft angle may necessitate varus osteotomy. If femoral version is normal or low, the proximal hamstring tendon is normal, and there are sciatic and/or posterior femoral cutaneous nerve symptoms secondary to lesser trochanteric IFI, then a lesser trochanterplasty may be considered, generating up to 10 mm of coronal plane ischiofemoral space opening. The latter, if performed without an iliopsoas repair, may be prone to iliopsoas atrophy and hip flexion weakness. If there is a proximal hamstring tendon tear, then ischioplasty may be considered. The latter can gain 5 to 7 mm of coronal plane ischiofemoral opening (**Fig. 6**A, B) with hamstring repair. The risk is ischial stress-related

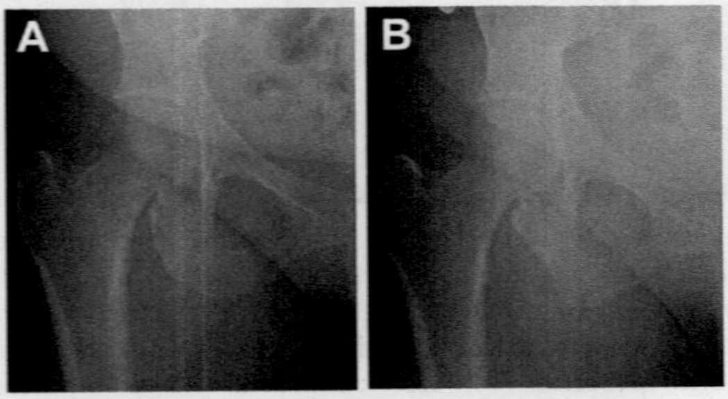

Fig. 6. (*A*) Anteroposterior pelvis plain radiograph in a 52 year old woman with severe pain secondary to ischiofemoral impingement from the lesser trochanter and a near full-thickness proximal hamstring tear; (*B*) same patient as in A, following open ischioplasty and proximal hamstring suture anchor repair.

bone injury if too much bone is removed, in addition to insufficient bone to support suture anchor hamstring repair. One of the pillars of deep gluteal surgical treatment involves sciatic and posterior femoral cutaneous neurolyses. This can be accomplished with endoscopic or open approaches.

Endoscopy of the deep gluteal space involves initial gluteal crease portal placement (medial, middle/central, lateral), with proximal and distal extension possible with accessory portal placement. Prone or lateral patient positioning has their own inherent advantages and disadvantages. The author prefers a prone approach for most deep gluteal space endoscopy. Endoscopy has a large advantage over open surgery due to less surgical dissection scar postoperatively. In addition, the scope permits high quality visualization of neurovascular structures without 1 or 2 surgical assistants retracting the gluteus maximus, often resulting in fatigue and poor visualization due to retractor placement. In addition, aberrant retractor placement proximally and medially may cause inadvertent pudendal nerve injury. Analogous to endoscopic versus open gluteus medius surgery, deep gluteal space endoscopy likely has a significantly lower postoperative infection risk. Endoscopy does have a potential risk of fluid extravasation into the pelvis and abdomen via the retroperitoneal space across the greater sciatic foramen, especially with proximal endoscopy above the obturator internus along the piriformis. Piriformis release must take great care in keep fluid pump pressure low and avoidance of iatrogenic neurovascular injury. Endoscopic release of fibrous/fibrovascular/vascular bands must ensure bands are not normal anatomy—inferior gluteal nerve/artery/vein and medial femoral circumflex artery are 2 common proximate structures that must be surgically respected. For vascular structures, intraoperative indocyanine green dye use via peripheral intravenous line can clearly elucidate vascularity for improved safety during both endoscopic and open surgery (**Fig. 7**A–C). Dynamic arthroscopic and fluoroscopic examination (**Fig. 8**) permits assessment of IFI from both lesser (extension, adduction, and external rotation) and greater (flexion, abduction, and external rotation) trochanters. Since normal sciatic nerve excursion should be up to 2.5 to 3.0 cm, neurolysis involves careful coagulation (for fibrovascular or vascular bands) and release of restrictive bands. As neurolysis progresses distally, hamstring muscle innervation branches must be carefully distinguished from pathologic bands. In open surgery, nerve stimulation instruments (CHECKPOINT Nerve Stimulator) and/or nerve monitoring may be highly

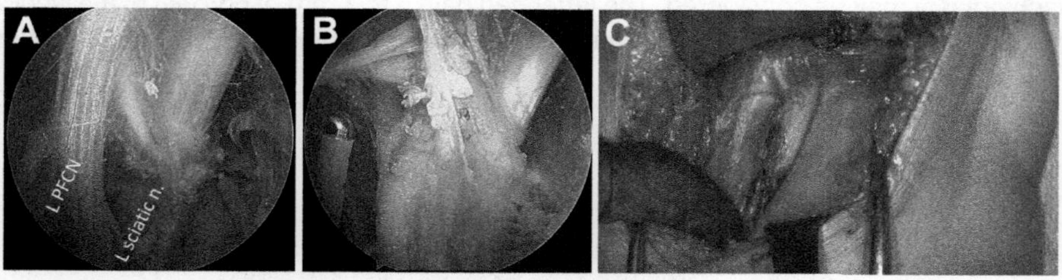

Fig. 7. (*A*) Left deep gluteal space endoscopy in a 44 year old woman demonstrating posterior femoral cutaneous and sciatic nerves, and a normal vascular conduit between nerves illuminated via intravenous ICG (indocyanine green) dye; (*B*) left deep gluteal space endoscopy in a 52 year old man after previous endoscopic hamstring repair and persistent postoperative sciatic and posterior femoral cutaneous nerve symptoms, demonstrating multiple perineural fibrous and fibrovascular bands; (*C*) open left proximal hamstring repair in a 55 year old man demonstrating 2 transverse perineural (posterior femoral cutaneous) vascular bands superficial to the sciatic nerve and lateral to the proximal hamstring (broad *green color* muscle).

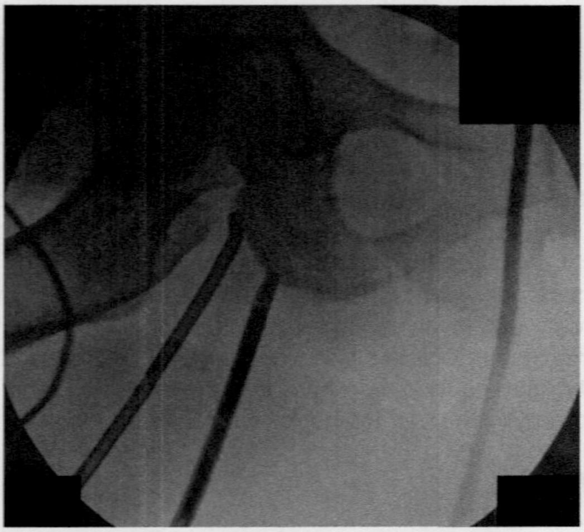

Fig. 8. Intraoperative fluoroscopic image of left greater trochanter—ischium ischiofemoral impingement in a 38 year old man at the proximal margin of the proximal hamstring tendon junction with the inferior margin of the obturator internus as it turns around from within the pelvis around the ischium to the deep gluteal space. This is the most common location of greater trochanter—ischium ischiofemoral impingement.

advantageous. Unfortunately, nerve stimulation instruments do not yet exist for endoscopic use. During surgery, as long as not contraindicated, intravenous tranexamic acid may reduce intraoperative and postoperative bleeding and a reduction in postoperative adhesions.

Following surgery, crutch-assisted ambulation should progress to weight bearing as tolerated without any gait abnormality (especially Trendelenburg) before crutch cessation. After isolated neurolysis without any hamstring repair or osteotomy/osteoplasty, this may variably take 2 to 4 weeks. Following surgery, structured personalized physical therapy should include early nerve glides to prevent nerve (both sciatic and posterior femoral cutaneous) tethering to surrounding structures. Nerve glides should always feel little (mild) to no symptoms—the nerve is gliding, not stretching; it is moving back and forth without tension, hence the name sometimes given nerve “flossing”. While being seated, and a slight slouch/arch in the low back, the knee should straighten/extend while looking up (neck extension) and the toes point straight out away from the body (ankle plantarflexion); then the knee should bend/flex while looking down “chin tuck” (neck flexion) and the toes pull up (ankle dorsiflexion). Postoperative oral losartan may reduce soft tissue adhesions, as has been used for hip arthroscopy in the central and peripheral compartments of the hip joint.[21] Following surgery, especially one that necessitates strength as a vital component of the recovery, proper nutrition (especially optimal protein intake—1.0–1.5 mg protein per pound body weight per day) is required. Without strong compelling evidence in the literature, nerve supplements may be offered postoperatively—alpha lipoic acid, omega-3’s, acetyl-L-carnitine, and vitamin C/B1/B12 (avoid high-dose vitamin B6, as this can worsen nerve symptoms).

SUMMARY

The deep gluteal space is a complex anatomic region associated with posterior hip symptoms. Pain is often longstanding due to challenges in diagnosis and treatment.

Individuals often receive conflicting, overlapping, and inaccurate diagnoses, and attempt multiple treatments, both nonsurgical and surgical, before ever receiving the correct diagnosis of deep gluteal syndrome. The clinical presentation involves symptoms and signs attributable to the deep gluteal space itself, in addition to the hip joint, peritrochanteric lateral hip, within the pelvis, and the lumbosacral spine. Imaging involves both 2 and 3 dimensional static modalities (plain radiographs, MRI, and CT). Collision-detection software may be valuable for dynamic osseous structural evaluation of the femur, ischium/pelvis, and lumbosacral spine/spinopelvic relationships. Nonsurgical treatment involves education-driven activity modification and personalized physical therapy, combined with oral medications and selective injections. Surgical treatment involves endoscopic or open management of the deep gluteal space, performed in isolation or combination with other hip procedures (eg, total hip arthroplasty, gluteus medius repair, lesser trochanterplasty, ischioplasty, and derotational osteotomy) either simultaneously or in staged fashion.

CLINICS CARE POINTS

- The etiology of pain in patients with deep gluteal space symptoms may be the deep gluteal space itself, the hip joint, lumbosacral spine, pelvis and pelvic floor, and the lateral hip, in isolation, or in combination.
- Accurate diagnosis of patients with pain emanating from the deep gluteal space requires thoughtful analysis of clinical presentation and imaging.
- Accurate and precise injections are vital to diagnosis and management of patients with pain in the deep gluteal space, including the ischiofemoral space itself, quadratus femoris, obturator internus, piriformis, sacroiliac joint, lumbosacral spine, hip joint, and lateral hip.
- Imaging workup for patients with pain in the deep gluteal space includes plain radiographs of the pelvis and hip, MRI (including neurography) of the pelvis and lumbosacral spine, and CT of the pelvis (including version analysis and 3D reconstruction, with dynamic collision detection as available, software permitting) with the feet positioned as in mid-stance phase of gait.
- Surgical treatment for patients with pain from the deep gluteal space includes a variety of endoscopic and open approaches, performed either in isolation or in combination, either simultaneously or in staged fashion.

DISCLOSURES

This investigation received no external or internal funding for this original research investigation. J.D. Harris is a paid consultant for Smith and Nephew; has received research support from Houston Methodist Hospital, Houston Texans; has received publication royalties from SLACK, Inc., and Thieme, Inc.; is on the Editorial Board of Arthroscopy: The Journal of Arthroscopic and Related Surgery; is on Committees for ISAKOS (International Society of Arthroscopy, Knee Surgery and Orthopedic Sports Medicine), ISHA (International Society of Hip Arthroscopy: The Hip Preservation Society).

REFERENCES

1. McCrory P, Bell S. Nerve entrapment syndromes as a cause of pain in the hip, groin and buttock. Sports Med 1999;27(4):261–74.

2. Beaton L, Anson B. The relation of the sciatic nerve and of its subdivisions to the piriformis muscle. Anat Rec 1937;70(1):1–5.
3. Smoll NR. Variations of the piriformis and sciatic nerve with clinical consequence: a review. Clin Anat 2010;23(1):8–17.
4. Martin HD, Shears SA, Johnson JC, et al. The endoscopic treatment of sciatic nerve entrapment/deep gluteal syndrome. Arthroscopy 2011;27(2):172–81.
5. Sunderland S, Hughes ES. Metrical and non-metrical features of the muscular branches of the sciatic nerve and its medial and lateral popliteal divisions. J Comp Neurol 1946;85(2):205–22.
6. Seidel PM, Seidel GK, Gans BM, et al. Precise localization of the motor nerve branches to the hamstring muscles: an aid to the conduct of neurolytic procedures. Arch Phys Med Rehabil 1996;77(11):1157–60.
7. Kizaki K, Uchida S, Shanmugaraj A, et al. Deep gluteal syndrome is defined as a non-discogenic sciatic nerve disorder with entrapment in the deep gluteal space: a systematic review. Knee Surg Sports Traumatol Arthrosc 2020;28-(10):3354–64.
8. Yeoman W. The relation of arthritis of the sacro-iliac joint to sciatica, with an analysis of 100 cases. Lancet (London, England) 1928;212(5492):1119–23.
9. Robinson DR. Pyriformis syndrome in relation to sciatic pain. Am J Surg 1947; 73(3):355–8.
10. Freynhagen R, Baron R, Gockel U, et al. painDETECT: a new screening questionnaire to identify neuropathic components in patients with back pain. Curr Med Res Opin 2006;22(10):1911–20.
11. Nakawaki M, Fukushima K, Inoue G, et al. Use of the painDETECT questionnaire to differentiate the nature of hip pain associated with a labrum tear. Asia Pac J Sports Med Arthrosc Rehabil Technol 2018;11:1–5.
12. DiSciullo AA, Stelzer JW, Martin SD. Dynamic ischiofemoral impingement: case-based evidence of progressive pathophysiology from hip abductor insufficiency: a report of two cases. JBJS case connector 2018;8(4):e107. https://doi.org/10.2106/jbjs.cc.18.00153.
13. Kivlan BR, Martin RL, Martin HD. Ischiofemoral impingement: defining the lesser trochanter-ischial space. Knee Surg Sports Traumatol Arthrosc 2017;25(1):72–6.
14. Harris JD. Editorial commentary: the pelvis is the lowest vertebral level: diagnostic approach to hip-spine syndrome. Arthroscopy 2022;38(10):2939–41.
15. Offierski CM, MacNab I. Hip-spine syndrome. Spine 1983;8(3):316–21.
16. Lerch TD, Boschung A, Leibold C, et al. Less in-toeing after femoral derotation osteotomy in adult patients with increased femoral version and posterior hip impingement compared to patients with femoral retroversion. Journal of hip preservation surgery 2022;9(1):35–43.
17. Lerch TD, Eichelberger P, Baur H, et al. Prevalence and diagnostic accuracy of in-toeing and out-toeing of the foot for patients with abnormal femoral torsion and femoroacetabular impingement: implications for hip arthroscopy and femoral derotation osteotomy. Bone Jt J 2019;101-b(10):1218–29.
18. Kivlan BR, Martin RL, Martin HD. Defining the greater trochanter-ischial space: a potential source of extra-articular impingement in the posterior hip region. Journal of hip preservation surgery 2016;3(4):352–7.
19. Gomez-Hoyos J, Khoury A, Schroder R, et al. The hip-spine effect: a biomechanical study of ischiofemoral impingement effect on lumbar facet joints. Arthroscopy 2017;33(1):101–7.

20. Bogunovic L, Lee SX, Haro MS, et al. Application of the goutallier/fuchs rotator cuff classification to the evaluation of hip abductor tendon tears and the clinical correlation with outcome after repair. Arthroscopy 2015;31(11):2145–51.
21. Philippon MJ, Ryan M, Martin MB, et al. Capsulolabral adhesions after hip arthroscopy for the treatment of femoroacetabular impingement: strategies during rehabilitation and return to sport to reduce the risk of revision. Arthroscopy, sports medicine, and rehabilitation 2022;4(1):e255–62.

Complications of Hip Arthroscopy: Prevention, Early Detection, and Management

Neel Badhe, BA[a], Vikas Khanduja, MA (Cantab), MB BS, MSc, FRCS (Tr & Orth), PhD[b,c,*]

KEYWORDS

• Hip arthroscopy • Complications • Prevention • Early detection • Management
• Nerve injury: fluid extravasation • Heterotopic ossification

KEY POINTS

- Hip arthroscopy, while minimally invasive, carries a spectrum of complications—from minor (temporary neuropraxia, chondrolabral injury, adhesions, hypothermia) to major (avascular necrosis, femoral neck fracture, infection, hip instability, thromboembolism)—with overall incidence influenced by surgeon experience and technical precision.
- Meticulous surgical technique is essential: accurate portal placement, controlled traction, capsular preservation, and careful labral handling reduce the risk of iatrogenic injury, nerve damage, instability, chondrolabral damage, and perineal complications.
- Prophylaxis and intra-operative measures: mechanical and pharmacological strategies mitigate risks of VTE, infection, heterotopic ossification, and adhesions; warm irrigation fluids and core temperature monitoring prevent hypothermia.
- Early recognition and monitoring: continuous intra-operative surveillance, structured post-operative follow-up, and vigilance for red-flag symptoms (neurological deficits, persistent pain, instability, swelling, erythema) enable timely intervention and optimize outcomes.
- Patient education and post-operative care are critical: counseling on weight-bearing restrictions, activity modification, signs of complications, and adherence to rehabilitation protocols improves recovery and helps prevent stress fractures, revision surgery, and other delayed complications.

[a] School of Clinical Medicine, University of Cambridge, Cambridge, UK; [b] Department of Trauma and Orthopaedic Surgery, Addenbrookes – Cambridge University Hospitals NHS Foundation Trust, University of Cambridge, Cambridge, UK; [c] Royal College of Surgeons of England
* Corresponding author. Department of Trauma and Orthopaedic Surgery, Addenbrookes –Cambridge University Hospitals NHS Foundation Trust, University of Cambridge, Cambridge, UK.
E-mail address: vk279@cam.ac.uk

Clin Sports Med 45 (2026) 735–752
https://doi.org/10.1016/j.csm.2026.04.003 sportsmed.theclinics.com

Abbreviations	
AVN	avascular necrosis
DVT	deep vein thrombosis
FAI	femoroacetabular impingement
HO	heterotopic ossification
MFCA	medial femoral circumflex artery
PE	pulmonary embolism
ROM	range of motion

INTRODUCTION

Hip arthroscopy has evolved significantly since the first cadaveric hip arthroscopy performed by Burman in 1931 and has experienced exponential interest and growth since the beginning of the 21st century.[1] A retrospective analysis of 3 US centers by Conyer and colleagues found that the mean number of hip arthroscopy procedures increased from 3.2 per year between 1988 and 2008 to 285.9 per year between 2016 and 2022.[2] These trends have also been observed in other health care systems around the world as well. A 727% increase in the number of hip arthroscopy procedures performed in NHS hospitals in England was reported between 2002 and 2013.[3] The rising popularity of hip arthroscopy is likely due to the shorter in-hospital stay, recovery period, less complications and its significant economic benefit.[4] Cost-effective analysis conducted by Mather and colleagues demonstrated that hip arthroscopy procedures, while associated with a higher initial cost, provided societal savings of $67,418 per patient compared with non-operative treatment and an additional 2.03 quality-adjusted life years over a 10 year period.[5,6]

However, despite being minimally invasive, hip arthroscopy is technically demanding and is associated with a steep learning curve, with studies suggesting that up to 520 cases may be required before complications are minimized.[7] Mehta and colleagues demonstrated that surgeon career volume was inversely correlated with risks of complications and reoperation rates.[8] These findings were supported by a systematic review conducted by Go and colleagues, who found that complication rates (0.5%–43.3% vs 0.5%–18.0%), revision arthroscopy rates (3.3%–10% vs 1.0%–4.2%), and conversion to total hip arthroplasty (12.2%–22.5% vs 1.5%–3.7%) all decreased with increasing surgical experience.[9] Notably, this trend persisted even among experienced surgeons, with high-volume surgeons (389–518 cases) experiencing a reoperation rate of 10.1%, compared with just 2.6% among the highest-volume surgeons ($\geq$519 cases).

Reported complication rates for hip arthroscopy vary significantly across the literature, ranging from 1.3% to 8.1%.[10–12] However, it is important to recognize that the figure of 8.1% reported by the systematic review conducted by Harris and colleagues excluded studies reporting no complications and most studies reported rates lie between 1.3% and 4.2%.[13–16] However, while complications are rare, there remains significant scope to reduce their incidence through prevention by improvements in both surgical technique and training.[17] Early detection and effective management are also essential for minimizing adverse outcomes and optimizing patient outcomes. This review aims to synthesize the current evidence on the major and minor complications associated with hip arthroscopy and outline strategies for their prevention, early detection, and management.

METHODS

A review of all peer-reviewed articles reporting on the prevention, early detection or management of complications following hip arthroscopy was conducted in October 2025 using the search strategy:

("hip arthroscopy" OR "arthroscopic hip surgery" OR "hip arthroscopic procedure*" OR "hip preservation") AND (complication* OR "adverse event*" OR reoperation* OR revision* "injur*" OR "infection" OR "fracture" OR "venous thromboembolism" OR VTE OR DVT OR PE OR "instability" OR "dislocation" OR "avascular necrosis" OR "heterotopic ossification" OR "adhesion*" OR "residual impingement" OR "inadequate resection") AND ("prevention" OR "prophylaxis" OR "risk reduction" OR "early detection" OR "screen*" OR "monitor*" OR "manage*" OR "treat*" OR "therap*" OR "intervention*").

Comprehensive searches of Medline, EMBASE and Cochrane CENTRAL databases were performed. Additional screening of the gray literature was conducted through bibliographic screening of previous review articles on this subject and Google Scholar. No restriction on study design was applied for inclusion. Animal studies, conference abstracts, and studies not published in the English language excluded.

CLASSIFICATION OF COMPLICATIONS

Complications following hip arthroscopy can be categorized by severity (major vs minor) or timing (intra-operative, early post-operative, late post-operative).[10,18] A summary of these complications and their incidence, as reported in the systematic review by Nakano and colleagues, is presented in **Table 1**.[10]

INTRAOPERATIVE COMPLICATIONS

Fluid Extravasation

Intra-abdominal fluid extravasation is the most frequently reported major complication of hip arthroscopy that is associated with extracapsular procedures involving iliopsoas tendon release, leakage through large capsulotomies, and prolonged operative times.[19,20] Fluid extravasation is serious and can result in abdominal compartment syndrome and potentially even cardiac arrest.[21] Due to the severity of these complications, risks of fluid extravasation should always be discussed with patients prior to undergoing hip arthroscopy procedures.[22]

Several precautions can be taken to minimize the risk of intra-abdominal fluid extravasation including keeping pump pressures below 50 mm Hg, performing iliopsoas tenotomies at the end of procedures, and reducing operative times.[18,23]

Table 1
Classification and incidence of complications following hip arthroscopy

	Major Complications		Minor Complications	
Timing	Complication	Incidence	Complication	Incidence
Intraoperative	Permanent	0.00%	Temporary nerve injury	0.9%
	nerve injury	0.04%	Iatrogenic chondral injury	0.4%
	Fluid extravasation		Iatrogenic labral injury	0.3%
			Hypothermia	0.01%
Early Post-operative	Deep infection	0.02%	Superficial infection	0.2%
	Pulmonary embolus	0.01%	Deep vein thrombosis	0.09%
	Hip instability	0.02%	Perineal skin damage	0.08%
	Hip dislocation	0.01%		
Late Post-operative	Avascular necrosis of	0.02%	Heterotopic ossification	0.6%
	the femoral head	0.03%	Adhesions	0.2%
	Neck of femur	0.01%		
	fracture			
	Death			

Additionally, this complication has been linked to arthroscopy undertaken following acute acetabular fractures and utmost care should be taken if performing a hip arthroscopy for this indication.[24,25]

The role of the anesthetist to prevent this complication cannot be underestimated. We recommend frequent abdominal palpation (every 30 minutes) and continuous intra-operative monitoring of airway pressures and vital signs for evidence of deterioration including hypotension, bradycardia, hypothermia, and especially increasing respiratory effort are essential to enable early detection and prompt intervention.[24,26,27] If suspected, diagnosis of abdominal fluid extravasation can be made with a CT or ultrasound, and immediate procedure abandonment and an urgent general surgical consult is essential.[18,19,22] Most cases resolve with supportive therapy including diuretics, maintenance of core body temperature, and frequent abdominal examinations and continuous monitoring of respiratory and cardiac function along with urine output.[28] Prolonged ventilation may be required in some cases until the fluid is reabsorbed and very rarely paracentesis or emergent decompressive laparotomy are indicated in cases of suspected abdominal compartment syndrome.[29]

Nerve Injury

Permanent motor nerve injury is a very rare complication of hip arthroscopy, with only one reported case in the literature.[10] However, the lateral femoral cutaneous nerve is at risk during supine hip arthroscopy and poor portal placement may result in injury. Because this nerve runs superficially, the skin incision should be kept superficial and should not extend unnecessarily into the subcutaneous fat. Careful identification of anatomic landmarks, meticulous dissection, and maintaining an appropriate distance from the expected nerve course during anterior portal placement are essential to prevent this complication. A cadaveric study by Bartlett and colleagues[30] demonstrated that relocating the anterior portal 5 mm medially or 15 mm laterally reduces the risk of lateral femoral cutaneous nerve injury.

While permanent nerve injury is rare, temporary neuropraxia is much more common, with the pudendal (0.3%), lateral femoral cutaneous (0.3%), and sciatic (0.2%) nerves most commonly affected.[10] A study by Telleria and colleagues found that maximum traction weight, rather than total traction time, was a greater predictor of post-procedural neuropraxia.[31] Consequently, the lowest amount of traction force necessary for adequate femoroacetabular distraction (typically 25–50 lbs for 8–10 mm of distraction) should be applied.[28,32] It has also been suggested that traction should not be applied continuously for a period of more than 2 hours to minimize the risk of neuropraxia.[33] Additionally, utilizing Trendelenburg positioning and padding the traction boot, bony prominences and the perineal post-adequately (>9 cm diameter) can help minimize the risk of compressive neuropraxia.[34,35] Ensuring that traction does not result in excessive genital pressure on the perineal post is also essential.[23]

More recently, post-less hip arthroscopy techniques have gained popularity as a means of reducing traction-related complications, particularly pudendal neuropraxia.[36] By eliminating the perineal post and utilizing patient positioning and friction to achieve distraction, these systems may reduce the risk of perineal compression while maintaining adequate joint access.

Postoperative manifestations of neuropraxia typically include transient numbness, paraesthesia, dysaesthesia, or, in the case of pudendal nerve involvement, perineal sensory disturbance or erectile dysfunction.[37] Most symptoms resolve spontaneously. In a prospective study by Dippmann and colleagues, neuropraxia-related symptoms were reported in 46% of patients at 6 weeks, decreasing to 18% at 1 year.[38] Management is usually conservative, consisting of observation, reassurance, and clinical follow-up. Persistent or progressive neurologic deficits may warrant further evaluation with imaging or electrodiagnostic studies.

Overall, careful attention to portal placement, traction management, patient positioning, and evolving techniques such as postless arthroscopy can further minimize the risk of nerve injury during hip arthroscopy.

Iatrogenic Chondrolabral Injury

Chondral and labral injury represents one of the most common minor complications of hip arthroscopy, with reported rates ranging from 0.7% to 20%.[39,40] These injuries most frequently occur during initial portal placement, when the spinal needle, guidewire, or trocar penetrates the acetabular labrum or contacts the femoral head cartilage during entry into the central compartment. Adequate joint distraction prior to portal creation, fluoroscopic guidance during needle advancement, and careful use of tactile feedback are important strategies to minimize this risk.[41] Domb and colleagues also suggested orienting the bevel of the spinal needle toward the femoral head during venting and subsequently toward the labrum once distraction is achieved to further reduce the risk of labral injury.[40] The senior author advocates insufflation of the hip joint with approximately 40 mL of normal saline before portal placement. This technique displaces the labrum away from the femoral head and enhances the fluoroscopic outline of the labrum, allowing the spinal needle to be directed safely beneath the labrum and thereby minimizing the risk of iatrogenic labral penetration.[42]

Limited visualization during arthroscopy is another important contributor to iatrogenic damage. Inadequate distraction, bleeding, capsular tightness, or poor portal trajectory can increase the likelihood of inadvertent cartilage contact by arthroscopic instruments. Chondral injury may occur during diagnostic arthroscopy, labral preparation, acetabular rim trimming, or femoral osteochondroplasty, particularly with the use of shavers, burrs, radiofrequency probes, or switching instruments.

Suboptimal suture anchor placement is also associated with chondrolabral injury. Anchors placed too close to the articular surface may penetrate the acetabular cartilage, while anchors positioned too medially may damage the labrum or enter the joint.[18] Matsuda and colleagues reported that anchor-related chondral injuries most commonly occur at the 1 o'clock position and when using anterior or mid-anterior portals.[43] Utilization of a distal anterolateral accessory portal can provide a safer trajectory for anchor insertion and reduce this risk.[44] Additional preventive strategies include the use of curved drill guides, smaller anchors, consideration of soft (ie, all suture) anchors, and careful control of drill depth.

The risk of iatrogenic injury may also be influenced by the surgical learning curve and procedural complexity. Meticulous technique, appropriate portal selection, and maintaining clear visualization throughout the procedure remain essential to minimize these complications.

Minor cartilage scuffing generally does not require intervention and rarely affects clinical outcomes. Badylak and Keene reported that iatrogenic labral injury did not significantly influence patient-reported outcomes at 2 year follow-up.[39]

Hypothermia

Hypothermia is defined as a reduction in core body temperature below 35 °C and is associated with increased bleeding, impaired tissue healing, and a higher risk of infection.[45–47] General anesthesia impairs thermoregulation and promotes peripheral vasodilation, leading to redistribution hypothermia, particularly during the early phase of surgery. In hip arthroscopy, the use of large volumes of irrigation fluid and prolonged exposure on the traction table may further exacerbate heat loss. A prospective study by Parodi and colleagues reported hypothermia in 2.7% of patients undergoing hip arthroscopy and identified prolonged operative time, low BMI, lower intra-operative blood pressure, and low irrigation fluid temperature as risk factors.[48] Preventive strategies include pre-operative warming, the use of warmed irrigation and intravenous fluids, forced-air warming blankets, and continuous core temperature monitoring.[49,50] Active warming should be instituted in affected patients postoperatively, with close monitoring for coagulopathy, delayed recovery, and infection.[50]

EARLY POST-OPERATIVE COMPLICATIONS

Infection

Compared with traditional open approaches, minimally invasive arthroscopic procedures are associated with a significantly reduced risk of infection. Despite this, deep infection and septic arthritis remain rare (0.02%), but important, complications to consider in patients undergoing hip arthroscopy.[10]

Reported risk factors include prolonged operative time, revision procedures, prior hip surgery, obesity, diabetes, and possibly intra-articular corticosteroid injections administered close to the time of surgery.[51,52]

It is essential to follow strict sterile technique. Additionally, while antibiotic prophylaxis in hip arthroscopy has not been closely studied, a systematic review and survey by Ekhtiari and colleagues found that routine prophylaxis was the most common practice in both the literature and among high-volume arthroscopy surgeons.[53]

Early diagnosis requires a high index of suspicion, as post-operative pain or swelling may initially obscure the clinical picture. Elevated inflammatory markers, including CRP and ESR, together with joint aspiration and microbiological analysis, can assist in confirming the diagnosis.[27]

Several cases of deep surgical site infections have been successfully managed with surgical drainage and intravenous antibiotics.[10] Although rare, septic arthritis following hip arthroscopy has also been reported.[54,55] Arthroscopic lavage has been shown to provide good outcomes in selected cases, with reduced morbidity and shorter hospital stay, although open irrigation and debridement continue to be considered the gold standard treatment in many cases.[56–59]

Superficial infection is a minor and relatively infrequent complication of hip arthroscopy, with an estimated incidence of 0.2%.[10] Again, maintaining diligent sterile technique minimizes the risk of these infections. Some studies have investigated the influence of prior intra-articular hip corticosteroid injections on the risk of post-operative infection in patients undergoing hip arthroscopy; however, this relationship remains unclear.[60–62] Patients should be educated to recognize early signs of infection, such as erythema and swelling.

Fortunately, when recognized early and treated promptly, the majority of infections following hip arthroscopy can be successfully managed without long-term sequelae.

Deep Vein Thrombosis and Pulmonary Embolism

Deep vein thrombosis (DVT) and pulmonary embolism (PE) are rare but potentially life-threatening complications of hip arthroscopy. While the estimated incidence of DVT following hip arthroscopy was estimated as 0.09% in a systematic review by Nakano and colleagues, a Doppler ultrasound study of 81 patients conducted by Salvo and colleagues found that 3 patients (3.7%) developed symptomatic DVT following hip arthroscopy.[18,63] While this study has a small sample size, it indicates these complications are generally underreported.

Recognized risk factors include prolonged operative or traction time, prior VTE, obesity, older age, hormonal therapy, and immobility. No formal guidelines currently exist for pharmacologic thromboprophylaxis in hip arthroscopy, though a 2024 Delphi study of 40 high-volume US arthroscopic hip surgeons found that 91.4% routinely use VTE prophylaxis, with 62.9% concerned that universal prophylaxis may increase bleeding or hemarthrosis.[64] A recent systematic review by Gao and colleagues concluded that high-risk patients should receive individualized pharmacologic prophylaxis, while standard-risk patients may not require routine anticoagulation.[65]

Mechanical prophylaxis, including intra-operative contralateral calf compression, below-knee elastic stockings, and early post-operative mobilization, remains recommended for all patients.[18,66] Prolonged traction and supine positioning may further predispose to venous stasis, highlighting the importance of intermittent limb mobilization during long procedures. Early recognition is critical: clinicians should monitor for unilateral leg swelling, pain, erythema, or sudden shortness of breath, and promptly initiate standard diagnostic workup and treatment if VTE is suspected. Overall, awareness of patient-specific and procedure-specific risk factors, combined with judicious prophylaxis and early mobilization, is essential to prevent these rare but serious complications.

Hip Instability and Dislocation

Iatrogenic hip instability and dislocation are well-documented but rare complications of hip arthroscopy. Key patient-related risk factors include hip dysplasia, generalized ligamentous laxity, female sex, prior hip surgery, connective tissue disorders, and early return to high-demand activity.[67–71] Most cases present within the early postoperative period, typically within the first 6 to 12 weeks.

Intra-operative causes of hip instability are summarized in **Table 2.**

Prevention strategies focus on preserving soft tissue stabilizers and restoring capsular integrity. These include: meticulous labral and ligamentum teres preservation, careful acetabular rim resection to maintain LCEA, minimizing unnecessary iliopsoas release, and avoiding large capsulotomies and if performed then routine capsular closure or plication, particularly in patients with ligamentous laxity, borderline dysplasia, or extensive capsulotomy. Capsular plication restores tension in the iliofemoral ligament and zona orbicularis, improving joint stability.[23]

Diagnosis and monitoring involve careful clinical assessment of anterior hip pain, giving-way episodes, or subluxation, supplemented where necessary by imaging,

Table 2
Iatrogenic structural causes of hip instability following hip arthroscopy

Structure	Function/Mechanism of Instability When Compromised
Ligamentum teres	Key stabilizing role in patients with mild dysplasia[72]
Iliopsoas tendon	Anterior dynamic stabilizer[73]
Acetabular labrum	Provides a suction-seal mechanism against distracting forces[74]
Proximal hip joint capsule and Zona orbicularis	Provides resistance to dislocation by forming a locking ring around the femoral neck[75]
Acetabular rim (overresection)	Excessive resection can create a dysplastic acetabulum with an LCEA <20°–25°, altering hip biomechanics, increasing reactive forces and chondrolabral degeneration[76]

including MRI or MR arthrography to evaluate capsular integrity, labral repair, and ligamentum teres injury. Dynamic fluoroscopy or stress radiographs may detect subtle subluxation in selected cases.

Management depends on severity. Mild post-arthroscopic instability may respond to activity modification, targeted physiotherapy, and bracing, whereas more severe or persistent cases require surgical intervention. Surgical strategies include arthroscopic or open capsular plication/reefing, labral repair or augmentation, and, in select cases, ligamentum teres reconstruction. Post-operative rehabilitation should emphasize controlled range of motion (ROM), gradual weight-bearing, and protection of repaired structures.[77–79]

Iatrogenic hip instability is rare but potentially debilitating. Prevention through preservation and repair of capsular and labral stabilizers, capsular plication in high-risk patients, and vigilant postoperative monitoring remains the cornerstone of management.

Perineal Skin Damage

Perineal skin injury is a recognized complication of hip arthroscopy, resulting from excessive pressure of the perineal post during traction. Most injuries are minor, presenting as localized edema, erythema, or small hematomas, but severe compression can result in pressure necrosis.[80–82] Risk is increased with prolonged traction, excessive force, inadequate padding, or incorrect post-positioning.

Prevention strategies mirror those used to reduce compressive neuropraxia. The perineal post should be positioned against the medial thigh in abduction, avoiding direct pressure on the genitalia or groin crease, allowing it to act as a lever rather than a point of compression.[83,84] Adequate padding (diameter >9 cm), limiting traction duration, and applying the lowest traction force necessary for adequate joint distraction further reduce the risk.[18]

Management is typically conservative, with spontaneous resolution in most cases through supportive care, including topical dressings and monitoring for tissue breakdown. Rarely, severe necrosis may require surgical debridement or reconstructive intervention. Early recognition and careful intraoperative positioning remain essential to prevent these potentially avoidable complications.

Preoperative skin assessment for patients with fragile skin, diabetes, or peripheral vascular disease may further identify those at higher risk, and postoperatively, patients should be educated to report persistent pain, blistering, or skin discoloration promptly.

Consideration of post-free distraction can also help in avoiding perineal skin damage as this risk has been generally negated by the use of the postless hip arthroscopy systems.[34,85,86]

LATE POSTOPERATIVE COMPLICATIONS

Avascular Necrosis of the Femoral Head

Avascular necrosis (AVN) of the femoral head is a rare but potentially devastating complication of hip arthroscopy.[12] Proposed contributing factors include excessive joint distraction, prolonged traction, elevated intra-articular pressure, partial capsulectomy, and iatrogenic injury to the femoral head blood supply, most commonly the lateral epiphyseal branch of the medial femoral circumflex artery (MFCA) during portal placement, capsulotomy, or femoral osteochondroplasty.[18,27]

Prevention strategies rely on a thorough understanding of the vascular anatomy and careful surgical technique. Surgeons should respect key anatomic landmarks, particularly the lateral synovial fold, which reliably delineates the lateral MFCA branches.[87] Femoral osteochondroplasty for cam-type femoroacetabular impingement (FAI) should terminate laterally before this fold to minimize vascular risk.[35] Avoiding release of the psoas tendon through the middle third of the capsule, where it lies in close proximity to the MFCA, further reduces the risk of direct arterial injury.[88] Additional preventive measures include limiting traction duration and force, using the lowest effective intra-articular fluid pressure, and minimizing unnecessary capsular disruption.[23]

Diagnosis and early detection are critical due to the often subtle early presentation. Persistent postoperative pain or functional limitation should prompt evaluation with magnetic resonance imaging (MRI), as radiographs may not reveal early AVN changes.[89] Early diagnosis may allow intervention with core decompression to preserve the femoral head, whereas more advanced or symptomatic cases generally require total hip arthroplasty.[90]

Patients with pre-existing vascular compromise, steroid use, alcohol excess, or previous hip surgery may have increased susceptibility and warrant heightened vigilance. Early recognition, conservative intra-operative management, and careful post-operative monitoring are central to minimizing the incidence and impact of this complication.

Neck of Femur Fracture

Femoral neck stress fractures are rare but serious complications of hip arthroscopy, associated with significant morbidity despite an estimated incidence of only 0.03%.[10] These fractures most commonly occur following femoral osteochondroplasty, particularly when excessive bone is resected, compromising the structural integrity of the proximal femur.

A cadaveric study by Mardones and colleagues demonstrated that up to 30% of femoral neck volume can be safely resected without significantly affecting load-bearing strength.[91] However, the same study found that even a 30% resection reduces the energy required to cause a fracture by 20%, highlighting the need to avoid over-resection and to respect femoral neck contours during osteochondroplasty.

Patient-related factors also contribute to fracture risk. Ayeni and colleagues reported a case of a non-displaced subcapital femoral neck fracture 5 weeks postoperatively, in a patient who had engaged in aggressive weight-bearing activity contrary to recommendations.[23,92,93] This underscores the importance of postoperative counseling and adherence to restricted weight-bearing protocols, particularly during the early healing phase.

Femoral neck stress fractures may be occult on standard radiographs, making MRI the modality of choice for early detection and accurate assessment.[94]

Treatment typically involves internal fixation, with careful monitoring for complications such as non-union or progression to displacement. In cases complicated by AVN of the femoral head, total hip arthroplasty may be indicated. Early recognition, careful surgical technique, and patient adherence to rehabilitation protocols are essential to minimize morbidity and optimize outcomes.

Inadequate Resection/Residual Impingement

Inadequate excision of cam or pincer lesions during hip arthroscopy is a recognized cause of persistent FAI and may necessitate revision surgery.[95] Residual impingement can lead to ongoing hip pain, limited ROM, and progression of chondrolabral damage despite technically successful initial surgery.[96]

Risk factors for incomplete resection include suboptimal preoperative imaging, inaccurate intra-operative assessment of lesion size, or conservative resection to avoid iatrogenic femoral neck fracture or cartilage injury. Technical strategies such as intra-operative fluoroscopy, dynamic impingement testing, and 3D preoperative planning can reduce the risk of under-resection.[97–99]

Diagnosis is typically based on persistent postoperative symptoms corroborated by imaging, often requiring CT or MRI to assess residual bony impingement. Management usually involves revision hip arthroscopy with targeted resection of the remaining cam or pincer lesion.[100] Careful surgical planning, including evaluation of joint space, cartilage status, and labral integrity, is essential to optimize outcomes and minimize the risk of further complications.

Heterotopic Ossification

Heterotopic ossification (HO) is a diverse pathologic process, defined as the formation of aberrant, mature lamellar bone in non-osseous tissue, and is one of the most frequent complications following arthroscopic hip procedures.[101] Early studies suggested that capsulectomy and unrepaired capsulotomy increase HO risk; however, more recent studies did not identify this association.[102,103] It has also been suggested that surgical trauma to the gluteal muscles and bone debris may trigger the development of HO; it is therefore important to lavage the hip carefully at the end of procedures to clear all debris from the joint.[18] A recent systematic review by Dean and colleagues[104] also demonstrated that secondary pharmacological HO prophylaxis with NSAIDs is effective in decreasing the risk of HO.

While some patients may present with localized pain, decreased ROM, impingement or instability, most patients with HO are asymptomatic, and HO is an incidental finding on postoperative radiographs.[105,106] Patients with HO on the first postoperative radiograph should receive ROM and radiographic follow-up for up to 12 months.[18] Management of HO is typically conservative with physical therapy and ROM exercises. Open or arthroscopic HO excision is patient-specific and can be considered in patients with refractory pain or significantly restricted ROM; however, surgery should only occur after HO maturity to minimize recurrence.[27,103,107]

Adhesions

Adhesions are a common cause of persistent symptoms and revision surgery following primary hip arthroscopy.[10,108] They typically form between the outer labral surface and the joint capsule after labral repair or rim recession, or between the femoral neck and capsule following osteochondroplasty.[18,109] These adhesions can disrupt the labral suction seal or mechanically impinge against the labrum, resulting in persistent stiffness, groin pain, and restricted hip flexion and rotation.[110]

Prevention strategies include mechanical prophylaxis such as continuous passive motion and early postoperative range-of-motion exercises, alongside chemoprophylaxis with anti-fibrotic agents or platelet-rich plasma in selected cases.[108,111,112]

Diagnosis remains challenging. MR arthrography is the most useful imaging modality, but a high index of clinical suspicion is often required, as radiographic findings may be subtle or inconclusive.[18] A recent systematic review by Keogh and colleagues highlighted that intra-operative identification during revision hip arthroscopy remains the most frequent method for diagnosing adhesions.[113]

Management typically involves adhesion lysis via revision arthroscopy, which has been shown to provide satisfactory short-term clinical outcomes. However, evidence regarding mid-to long-term efficacy remains limited, underscoring the need for further research into optimal strategies for prevention and management.

SUMMARY

Hip arthroscopy has rapidly evolved to become a cornerstone of modern orthopedic surgery. Although minimally invasive, it remains technically demanding with a steep learning curve, and carries an inherent risk of complications, with reported rates ranging from 1.3% to 4.2%, influenced by surgeon experience.

Complications can be classified by severity (major vs minor) and timing (intra-operative, early post-operative, late post-operative). Major complications include fluid extravasation, permanent nerve injury, deep infection, venous thromboembolism, hip instability, AVN of the femoral head, femoral neck fractures, and rarely, death. Minor complications include temporary neuropraxia, chondrolabral injury, inadequate resection requiring revision, hypothermia, superficial infection, HO, adhesions, and perineal skin damage.

Prevention strategies focus on meticulous surgical technique: accurate positioning, controlled traction, careful portal placement, preservation of soft tissue stabilizers, thorough lavage, and respect for vascular anatomy. Mechanical and pharmacologic prophylaxis are essential for venous thromboembolism, infection, HO, and adhesions.

Early detection and timely intervention are critical to optimize outcomes. This is facilitated by intra-operative monitoring, patient education, structured post-operative follow-up, and appropriate imaging such as MRI or MR arthrography when indicated. By combining preventive measures, vigilance, and evidence-based management, hip arthroscopy can be performed safely while maximizing functional recovery and minimizing adverse events.

CLINICS CARE POINTS

- Continuous intra-operative monitoring of vital signs, fluid balance, and limb perfusion is essential for early detection of fluid extravasation, abdominal compartment syndrome, hemodynamic instability, and neuropraxia, enabling urgent intervention when required.
- Reducing operative time, maintaining low irrigation pump pressures, minimizing traction force and duration, and ensuring adequate perineal post-padding help reduce the risk of fluid extravasation, neuropraxia, and perineal skin injury. Post-less hip arthroscopy techniques may further reduce perineal complications and traction-related nerve injury.
- Accurate portal placement and careful soft tissue handling are critical to prevent chondrolabral injury, labral puncture, nerve injury, and iatrogenic hip instability. Techniques such as joint distension with saline to visualize the labrum can help avoid labral puncture.
- Thorough understanding of hip vascular anatomy and careful respect for anatomical landmarks reduce the risk of AVN of the femoral head during capsulotomy or femoral osteochondroplasty.
- Avoid over-resection of femoral neck or acetabular rim, and provide patients with post-operative weight-bearing restrictions, to minimize the risk of femoral neck stress fractures and residual cam/pincer lesions requiring revision surgery.
- Capsular preservation, plication, and careful labral repair help prevent post-operative hip instability, particularly in patients with ligamentous laxity or dysplasia.
- Mechanical and pharmacological prophylaxis should be considered to mitigate venous thromboembolism, infection, HO, and adhesion formation. Early mobilization, compression stockings, and judicious NSAID use are key adjuncts.
- Temperature management with warmed irrigation fluids, active warming blankets, and monitoring of core temperature helps prevent intraoperative and postoperative hypothermia, which can increase bleeding and infection risk.
- Early recognition of red-flag symptoms—including persistent neurological deficits, groin pain, hip instability, erythema, swelling, or unexplained post-operative pain—is critical to initiate appropriate imaging, diagnosis, and timely intervention.
- Structured post-operative follow-up and patient education regarding signs of infection, VTE, neuropraxia, HO, adhesions, or instability improve early detection and management of complications.

- Meticulous joint lavage at the end of the procedure reduces HO risk, while controlled traction, proper portal placement, and careful labral handling limit adhesion formation.
- Consider revision surgery only after thorough assessment in patients with persistent symptoms from adhesions, HO, or inadequate resection, using MRI, MR arthrography, or other imaging as indicated.

DISCLOSURES

The authors have nothing to disclose.

REFERENCES

1. Burman MS. Arthroscopy or the direct visualization of joints: an experimental cadaver study. JBJS 1931;13(4):669–95.
2. Conyer RT, Cleary EJ, Wang AS, et al. A multicenter analysis of 3 decades of hip arthroscopy: evolving techniques and growing patient volumes from 1988 to 2022. Orthop J Sports Med 2024;12(10):23259671241277793. https://doi.org/10.1177/23259671241277793.
3. Palmer AJ, Malak TT, Broomfield J, et al. Past and projected temporal trends in arthroscopic hip surgery in England between 2002 and 2013. BMJ Open Sport Exerc Med 2016;2(1):e000082. https://doi.org/10.1136/bmjsem-2015-000082.
4. Addai D, Zarkos J, Pettit M, et al. Outcomes following surgical management of femoroacetabular impingement: a systematic review and meta-analysis of different surgical techniques. Bone Joint Res 2021;10(9):574–90.
5. Mather RC, Nho SJ, Federer A, et al. Effects of arthroscopy for femoroacetabular impingement syndrome on quality of life and economic outcomes. Am J Sports Med 2018;46(5):1205–13.
6. Go CC, Kyin C, Chen JW, et al. Cost-effectiveness of hip arthroscopy for treatment of femoroacetabular impingement syndrome and labral tears: a systematic review. Orthop J Sports Med 2021;9(3):2325967120987538. https://doi.org/10.1177/2325967120987538.
7. Almasri M, Ayeni OR. Editorial commentary: defining proficiency in hip arthroscopic surgery is facing its own learning curve. Arthroscopy 2020;36(12):3106–7.
8. Mehta N, Chamberlin P, Marx RG, et al. Defining the learning curve for hip arthroscopy: a threshold analysis of the volume-outcomes relationship. Am J Sports Med 2018;46(6):1284–93.
9. Go CC, Kyin C, Maldonado DR, et al. Surgeon experience in hip arthroscopy affects surgical time, complication rate, and reoperation rate: a systematic review on the learning curve. Arthroscopy 2020;36(12):3092–105.
10. Nakano N, Lisenda L, Jones TL, et al. Complications following arthroscopic surgery of the hip: a systematic review of 36 761 cases. Bone Jt J 2017;99-b(12):1577–83.
11. Byrd JW. Hip arthroscopy. The supine position. Clin Sports Med 2001;20(4):703–31.
12. Harris JD, McCormick FM, Abrams GD, et al. Complications and reoperations during and after hip arthroscopy: a systematic review of 92 studies and more than 6,000 patients. Arthroscopy 2013;29(3):589–95.
13. de Sa D, Stephens K, Parmar D, et al. A comparison of supine and lateral decubitus positions for hip arthroscopy: a systematic review of outcomes and complications. Arthroscopy 2016;32(4):716–25.e8.

14. Niroopan G, de Sa D, MacDonald A, et al. Hip arthroscopy in trauma: a systematic review of indications, efficacy, and complications. Arthroscopy 2016;32(4):692–703.e1.
15. Truntzer JN, Hoppe DJ, Shapiro LM, et al. Complication rates for hip arthroscopy are underestimated: a population-based study. Arthroscopy 2017;33(6):1194–201.
16. Cvetanovich GL, Chalmers PN, Levy DM, et al. Hip arthroscopy surgical volume trends and 30-day postoperative complications. Arthrosc J Arthrosc Relat Surg 2016;32(7):1286–92.
17. Brand JC, Rossi MJ, Lubowitz JH. Hip arthroscopy complications are rare, but there is room for improvement. Arthroscopy 2019;35(5):1297–9.
18. Nakano N, Khanduja V. Complications in hip arthroscopy. Muscles Ligaments Tendons J 2016;6(3):402–9.
19. Haupt U, Völkle D, Waldherr C, et al. Intra-and retroperitoneal irrigation liquid after arthroscopy of the hip joint. Arthrosc J Arthrosc Relat Surg 2008;24(8):966–8.
20. Verma M, Sekiya JK. Intrathoracic fluid extravasation after hip arthroscopy. Arthroscopy 2010;26(9 Suppl):S90–4.
21. Bartlett CS, DiFelice GS, Buly RL, et al. Cardiac arrest as a result of intraabdominal extravasation of fluid during arthroscopic removal of a loose body from the hip joint of a patient with an acetabular fracture. J Orthop Trauma 1998;12(4):294–9.
22. Ladner B, Nester K, Cascio B. Abdominal fluid extravasation during hip arthroscopy. Arthrosc J Arthrosc Relat Surg 2010;26(1):131–5.
23. Gupta A, Redmond JM, Hammarstedt JE, et al. Safety measures in hip arthroscopy and their efficacy in minimizing complications: a systematic review of the evidence. Arthroscopy 2014;30(10):1342–8.
24. Burrus MT, Cowan JB, Bedi A. Avoiding failure in hip arthroscopy: complications, pearls, and pitfalls. Clin Sports Med 2016;35(3):487–501.
25. Weber AE, Harris JD, Nho SJ. Complications in hip arthroscopy: a systematic review and strategies for prevention. Sports Med Arthrosc Rev 2015;23(4):187–93.
26. Ekhtiari S, Haldane CE, de Sa D, et al. Fluid extravasation in hip arthroscopy: a systematic review. Arthroscopy 2017;33(4):873–80.
27. Castro A, de Melo C, Leal F. Complications in hip arthroscopy: recognizing and managing adverse events. J Clin Orthop Trauma 2025;69:103144. https://doi.org/10.1016/j.jcot.2025.103144.
28. Fabricant PD, Maak TG, Cross MB, et al. Avoiding complications in hip arthroscopy. Operat Tech Sports Med 2011;19(2):108–13.
29. Ciemniewska-Gorzela K, Piontek T, Szulc A. Abdominal compartment syndrome–the prevention and treatment of possible lethal complications following hip arthroscopy: a case report. J Med Case Rep 2014;8:368.
30. Bartlett JD, Lawrence JE, Khanduja V. What is the risk posed to the lateral femoral cutaneous nerve during the use of the anterior portal of supine hip arthroscopy and the minimally invasive anterior approach for total hip arthroplasty? Arthroscopy 2018;34(6):1833–40.
31. Telleria JJ, Safran MR, Harris AH, et al. Risk of sciatic nerve traction injury during hip arthroscopy—is it the amount or duration? An intraoperative nerve monitoring study. J Bone Joint Surg Am 2012;94(22):2025–32.
32. Papavasiliou A, Bardakos N. Complications of arthroscopic surgery of the hip. Bone & Joint Research 2012;1(7):131–44.

33. Sampson TG. Complications of hip arthroscopy. Clin Sports Med 2001;20(4): 831–6.
34. Mei-Dan O, Kraeutler MJ, Garabekyan T, et al. Hip distraction without a perineal post: a prospective study of 1000 hip arthroscopy cases. Am J Sports Med 2018;46(3):632–41.
35. Ilizaliturri VM Jr. Complications of arthroscopic femoroacetabular impingement treatment: a review. Clin Orthop Relat Res 2009;467(3):760–8.
36. Moran J, Jimenez AE. Editorial commentary: postless hip arthroscopy may help optimize outcomes, but use of a post is acceptable and is indicated in select cases. Arthroscopy 2025;41(3):657–9.
37. Habib A, Haldane CE, Ekhtiari S, et al. Pudendal nerve injury is a relatively common but transient complication of hip arthroscopy. Knee Surg Sports Traumatol Arthrosc 2018;26(3):969–75.
38. Dippmann C, Thorborg K, Kraemer O, et al. Symptoms of nerve dysfunction after hip arthroscopy: an under-reported complication? Arthroscopy 2014;30(2):202–7.
39. Badylak JS, Keene JS. Do iatrogenic punctures of the labrum affect the clinical results of hip arthroscopy? Arthroscopy 2011;27(6):761–7.
40. Domb BG, Botser IB. Iatrogenic labral puncture of the hip is avoidable. Arthroscopy 2012;28(3):305–7 [author reply: 307-8].
41. Messer KP, Price AD, Kraeutler MJ. Step-by-step guide for safe joint access during hip arthroscopy. Arthrosc Tech 2025;14(6):103524. https://doi.org/10.1016/j.eats.2025.103524.
42. Sunil Kumar KH, Lisenda L, Khanduja V. Avoiding iatrogenic injury during portal placement in hip arthroscopy. Ann R Coll Surg Engl 2016;98(8):592–3.
43. Matsuda DK, Bharam S, White BJ, et al. Anchor-induced chondral damage in the hip. J Hip Preserv Surg 2015;2(1):56–64.
44. Stanton M, Banffy M. Safe angle of anchor insertion for labral repair during hip arthroscopy. Arthroscopy 2016;32(9):1793–7.
45. Duong H, Patel G. Hypothermia. StatPearls. StatPearls Publishing Copyright © 2025, StatPearls Publishing LLC.; 2025.
46. Torossian A. Thermal management during anaesthesia and thermoregulation standards for the prevention of inadvertent perioperative hypothermia. Best Pract Res Clin Anaesthesiol 2008;22(4):659–68.
47. Sessler DI. Complications and treatment of mild hypothermia. Anesthesiology 2001;95(2):531–43.
48. Parodi D, Tobar C, Valderrama J, et al. Hip arthroscopy and hypothermia. Arthroscopy 2012;28(7):924–8.
49. Suri TS, Sardesai A, Volpin A, et al. Incidence of hypothermia and factors affecting variation in core body temperature in patients undergoing arthroscopic surgery of the hip. Acta Orthop Belg 2019;85(4):535–9.
50. Sardesai A, Hujazi I, Khanduja V. Surgical access warming blanket to prevent hypothermia after hip arthroscopy. Arthroscopy 2012;28(8):1045–6.
51. Nian PP, Gordon AM, Baidya J, et al. Assessing the risk factors for surgical site and deep wound infections following hip arthroscopy: a nationwide study of 75,577 patients. J Am Acad Orthop Surg 2025;33(13):739–45.
52. Aamer S, Tokhi I, Asim M, et al. Postoperative infection following hip arthroscopy in patients receiving preoperative intra-articular injections: a systematic review and meta-analysis. Cureus 2024;16(6):e61649. https://doi.org/10.7759/cureus.61649.
53. Ekhtiari S, Haldane CE, de Sa D, et al. The use of antibiotic prophylaxis in hip arthroscopy is under-reported and lacks evidence-based guidelines: a systematic review and survey. Journal of ISAKOS 2018;3(2):105–9.

54. Seijas R, Ares O, Sallent A, et al. Hip arthroscopy complications regarding surgery and early postoperative care: retrospective study and review of literature. Musculoskelet Surg 2017;101(2):119–31.
55. Clarke M, Arora A, Villar R. Hip arthroscopy: complications in 1054 cases. Clin Orthop Relat Res 2003;406(1):84–8.
56. Kim SJ, Choi NH, Ko SH, et al. Arthroscopic treatment of septic arthritis of the hip. Clin Orthop Relat Res 2003;407:211–4.
57. Nusem I, Jabur MK, Playford EG. Arthroscopic treatment of septic arthritis of the hip. Arthroscopy 2006;22(8):902.e1–3.
58. Blitzer CM. Arthroscopic management of septic arthritis of the hip. Arthroscopy 1993;9(4):414–6.
59. Chung WK, Slater GL, Bates EH. Treatment of septic arthritis of the hip by arthroscopic lavage. J Pediatr Orthop 1993;13(4):444–6.
60. Byrd JWT, Bardowski EA, Civils AN, et al. The safety of hip arthroscopy within 3 months of an intra-articular injection. J Bone Joint Surg Am 2019;101(16): 1467–9.
61. Varady NH, Amen TB, Abraham PF, et al. Image-guided intra-articular hip injections and risk of infection after hip arthroscopy. Am J Sports Med 2021;49(9):2482–8.
62. Surucu S, Halperin SJ, Monahan PF, et al. Corticosteroid injections administered within 4 weeks prior to hip arthroscopy are associated with higher rates of postoperative infection. Arthroscopy 2024;40(9):2381–5.e1.
63. Salvo JP, Troxell CR, Duggan DP. Incidence of venous thromboembolic disease following hip arthroscopy. Orthopedics 2010;33(9):664.
64. Parsa A, Bedi A, Domb BG. Current trends for venous thromboembolic prophylaxis for hip arthroscopy: a modified Delphi and nominal group technique consensus study. J. Hip Preserv. Surg 2024;11(3):192–7.
65. Gao T, Lv K, Zhang H, et al. Venous thromboembolism after hip arthroscopy: a systematic review of incidence, risk factors, and international guidelines. Front Surg 2025;12:1658428. https://doi.org/10.3389/fsurg.2025.1658428.
66. Aali Rezaie A, Azboy I, Parvizi J. Venous thromboembolism prophylaxis after hip preservation surgery: a review and presentation of institutional experience. J Hip Preserv Surg 2018;5(3):181–9.
67. Yeung M, Memon M, Simunovic N, et al. Gross instability after hip arthroscopy: an analysis of case reports evaluating surgical and patient factors. Arthroscopy 2016;32(6):1196–204.e1.
68. Duplantier NL, McCulloch PC, Nho SJ, et al. Hip dislocation or subluxation after hip arthroscopy: a systematic review. Arthroscopy 2016;32(7):1428–34.
69. Matsuda DK. Acute iatrogenic dislocation following hip impingement arthroscopic surgery. Arthroscopy 2009;25(4):400–4.
70. Ranawat AS, McClincy M, Sekiya JK. Anterior dislocation of the hip after arthroscopy in a patient with capsular laxity of the hip: a case report. JBJS 2009;91(1): 192–7.
71. Wolf JM, Cannada L, Van Heest AE, et al. Male and female differences in musculoskeletal disease. J Am Acad Orthop Surg 2015;23(6):339–47.
72. Mei-Dan O, McConkey MO, Brick M. Catastrophic failure of hip arthroscopy due to iatrogenic instability: can partial division of the ligamentum teres and iliofemoral ligament cause subluxation? Arthroscopy 2012;28(3):440–5.
73. Fabricant PD, Bedi A, De La Torre K, et al. Clinical outcomes after arthroscopic psoas lengthening: the effect of femoral version. Arthroscopy 2012;28(7):965–71.

74. Storaci HW, Utsunomiya H, Kemler BR, et al. The hip suction seal, part i: the role of acetabular labral height on hip distractive stability. Am J Sports Med 2020;48(11):2726–32.
75. Ito H, Song Y, Lindsey DP, et al. The proximal hip joint capsule and the zona orbicularis contribute to hip joint stability in distraction. J Orthop Res 2009;27(8):989–95.
76. Bhatia S, Lee S, Shewman E, et al. Effects of acetabular rim trimming on hip joint contact pressures: how much is too much? Am J Sports Med 2015;43(9):2138–45.
77. Zárate Leal MF, Bautista M, Sánchez-Vergel A. Late post-arthroscopy hip instability. Diagnosis, treatment, and 5-year follow-up: a case report. Int J Surg Case Rep 2024;115:109323.
78. Yeung M, Khan M, Williams D, et al. Anterior hip capsuloligamentous reconstruction with achilles allograft following gross hip instability post-arthroscopy. Knee Surg Sports Traumatol Arthrosc 2017;25(1):3–8.
79. Gehrman M, Cornell M, Seeley M. Iatrogenic hip instability after hip arthroscopy: is there a role for open capsular reconstruction?: a case report. JBJS Case Connector 2019;9(2):e0091.
80. Funke EL, Munzinger U. Complications, in hip arthroscopy. Arthroscopy 1996;12(2):156–9.
81. Gedouin J-E, May O, Bonin N, et al. Assessment of arthroscopic management of femoroacetabular impingement. A prospective multicenter study. Orthop Traumatol 2010;96(8):S59–67.
82. Souza BG, Dani WS, Honda EK, et al. Do complications in hip arthroscopy change with experience? Arthroscopy 2010;26(8):1053–7.
83. Byrd JT. Hip arthroscopy: surgical indications. Arthroscopy 2006;22(12):1260–2.
84. Smart LR, Oetgen M, Noonan B, et al. Beginning hip arthroscopy: indications, positioning, portals, basic techniques, and complications. Arthroscopy 2007;23(12):1348–53.
85. Kraeutler MJ, Fasulo SM, Dávila Castrodad IM, et al. A prospective comparison of groin-related complications after hip arthroscopy with and without a perineal post. Am J Sports Med 2023;51(1):155–9.
86. Volpi A, Hopkins KT, McHugh M, et al. Physician reported outcomes of hip arthroscopy without a perineal post: an international survey. J. Hip Preserv. Surg 2024;11(1):3–7.
87. Gautier E, Ganz K, Krügel N, et al. Anatomy of the medial femoral circumflex artery and its surgical implications. J Bone Joint Surg Br 2000;82(5):679–83.
88. McCormick F, Kleweno CP, Kim YJ, et al. Vascular safe zones in hip arthroscopy. Am J Sports Med 2011;39(Suppl):64s–71s.
89. Stoica Z, Dumitrescu D, Popescu M, et al. Imaging of avascular necrosis of femoral head: familiar methods and newer trends. Curr Health Sci J 2009;35(1):23–8.
90. Hua K-c, Yang X-g, Feng J-t, et al. The efficacy and safety of core decompression for the treatment of femoral head necrosis: a systematic review and meta-analysis. J Orthop Surg Res 2019;14(1):306.
91. Mardones RM, Gonzalez C, Chen Q, et al. Surgical treatment of femoroacetabular impingement: evaluation of the effect of the size of the resection. J Bone Joint Surg Am 2005;87(2):273–9.

92. Ayeni OR, Bedi A, Lorich DG, et al. Femoral neck fracture after arthroscopic management of femoroacetabular impingement: a case report. J Bone Joint Surg Am 2011;93(9):e47.
93. Varshneya K, Abrams GD, Sherman SL, et al. Patient-specific risk factors exist for hip fractures after arthroscopic femoroacetabular impingement surgery, but not for dislocation-an analysis of more than 25,000 hip arthroscopies. Arthrosc Sports Med Rehabil 2022;4(2):e519–25.
94. Larson CM, Clohisy JC, Beaulé PE, et al. Intraoperative and early postoperative complications after hip arthroscopic surgery: a prospective multicenter trial utilizing a validated grading scheme. Am J Sports Med 2016;44(9):2292–8.
95. Sardana V, Philippon MJ, de Sa D, et al. Revision hip arthroscopy indications and outcomes: a systematic review. Arthroscopy 2015;31(10):2047–55.
96. Shin JJ, de Sa DL, Burnham JM, et al. Refractory pain following hip arthroscopy: evaluation and management. J Hip Preserv Surg 2018;5(1):3–14.
97. Zheng F, Daofeng W, Guanyang S, et al. Quantitative evaluation and preoperative planning using three-dimensional CT profiles improves the accuracy of bony correction under primary hip arthroscopy and clinical outcomes in the setting of cam-type femoroacetabular impingement syndrome. Orthop Surg 2025;17(8):2422–34.
98. Ross JR, Bedi A, Stone RM, et al. Intraoperative fluoroscopic imaging to treat cam deformities: correlation with 3-dimensional computed tomography. Am J Sports Med 2014;42(6):1370–6.
99. Locks R, Chahla J, Mitchell JJ, et al. Dynamic hip examination for assessment of impingement during hip arthroscopy. Arthrosc Tech 2016;5(6):e1367–72.
100. Ross JR, Larson CM, Adeoyo O, et al. Residual deformity is the most common reason for revision hip arthroscopy: a three-dimensional CT study. Clin Orthop Relat Res 2015;473(4):1388–95.
101. Meyers C, Lisiecki J, Miller S, et al. Heterotopic ossification: a comprehensive review. JBMR Plus 2019;3(4):e10172. https://doi.org/10.1002/jbm4.10172.
102. Beckmann JT, Wylie JD, Kapron AL, et al. The effect of NSAID prophylaxis and operative variables on heterotopic ossification after hip arthroscopy. Am J Sports Med 2014;42(6):1359–64.
103. Amar E, Warschawski Y, Sampson TG, et al. Capsular closure does not affect development of heterotopic ossification after hip arthroscopy. Arthroscopy 2015;31(2):225–30.
104. Dean RS, Hamama BA, Cavinatto L, et al. Chemoprophylaxis for heterotopic ossification following hip arthroscopy: a systematic review. J isakos 2023;8(6): 484–9.
105. Seijas R, Barastegui D, de Celis CL, et al. Heterotopic ossification in hip arthroscopy. Surg J 2023;9(01):e8–12.
106. Arshad Z, Maughan HD, Garner M, et al. Incidence of heterotopic ossification following hip arthroscopy is low: considerations for routine prophylaxis. Int Orthop 2022;46(7):1489–500.
107. Kurz AZ, LeRoux E, Riediger M, et al. Heterotopic ossification in hip arthroscopy: an updated review. Current Reviews in Musculoskeletal Medicine 2019; 12(2):147–55.
108. Willimon SC, Briggs KK, Philippon MJ. Intra-articular adhesions following hip arthroscopy: a risk factor analysis. Knee Surg Sports Traumatol Arthrosc 2014;22(4):822–5.

109. Krueger A, Leunig M, Siebenrock KA, et al. Hip arthroscopy after previous surgical hip dislocation for femoroacetabular impingement. Arthroscopy 2007;23-(12):1285–9.e1.
110. Ruzbarsky JJ, Soares RW, Comfort SM, et al. Adhesions in the setting of hip arthroscopy. EFORT Open Rev 2023;8(11):792–7.
111. Philippon MJ, Ryan M, Martin MB, et al. Capsulolabral adhesions after hip arthroscopy for the treatment of femoroacetabular impingement: strategies during rehabilitation and return to sport to reduce the risk of revision. Arthrosc Sports Med Rehabil 2022;4(1):e255–62.
112. Den Hartog TJ, Leary SM, Schaver AL, et al. The incidence and outcomes following treatment of capsulolabral adhesions in hip arthroscopy: a systematic review. Iowa Orthop J 2023;43(2):146–55.
113. Keogh JAJ, Keng I, Ifabiyi M, et al. Adhesions after hip arthroscopy are associated with revision but show poorly defined criteria for diagnosis and operative management: a systematic review. Arthroscopy 2025;41(4):1123–39.e1.

United States Postal Service

Statement of Ownership, Management and Circulation
(All Periodicals Publications Except Requester Publications)

1. Publication Title	2. Publication Number	3. Filing Date
CLINICS IN SPORTS MEDICINE	0 0 0 - 7 0 2	08/21/2026
4. Issue Frequency	**5. Number of Issues Published Annually**	**6. Annual Subscription Price**
JAN, APR, JUL, OCT	4	$399.00

7. Complete Mailing Address of Known Office of Publication (Not printer) (Street, city, county, state, and ZIP+4)
Addr 1: Elsevier INC
Addr 2: 230 Park Ave Ste 800
City, State ZIP: New York NY 10169

Contact Person: Mohana Priya Damodharan
Telephone: 91-44-4299-4077

8. Complete Mailing Address of Headquarters or General Business Office of Publisher (Not Printer)
Addr 1: Elsevier INC
Addr 2: 230 Park Ave Ste 800
City, State ZIP: New York NY 10169

9. Full Names and Complete Mailing Addresses of Publisher, Editor and Managing Editor (do not leave blank)

Publisher (Name and complete mailing address)
Name: Dolores Meloni, ELSEVIER INC.
Addr 1: 1600 JOHN F KENNEDY BLVD. SUITE 1600
Addr 2:
City, State ZIP: PHILADELPHIA, PA 19103-2899

Editor (Name and complete mailing address)
Name: ASHLIE JACKMAN, ELSEVIER INC.
Addr 1: 1ST FLOOR, NIELSEN HOUSE, JOHN SMITH DRIVE
Addr 2:
City, State ZIP: OXFORD, OX4 2WB, UK

Managing Editor (Name and complete mailing address)
Name: PATRICK MANLEY, ELSEVIER INC.
Addr 1: 1600 JOHN F KENNEDY BLVD. SUITE 1600
Addr 2:
City, State ZIP: PHILADELPHIA, PA 19103-2899

10. Owner (Do not leave blank. If the publication is owned by a corporation, give the name and address of the corporation immediately followed by the names and addresses of all stockholders owning or holding 1 Percent or more of the total amount of stock. If not owned by a corporation, give the names and addresses of all the individual owners. If owned by a partnership or other unincorporated firm, give it's name and address as well as those of each individual owner. If the publication is published by a nonprofit organization, give it's name and address.)

Full Name	Complete Mailing Address
WHOLLY OWNED SUBSIDIARY OF REED/ELSEVIER,	1600 JOHN F KENNEDY BLVD. SUITE 1600
US HOLDINGS	PHILADELPHIA, PA 19103-2899

11. Known Bondholders, Mortgagees and Other Security Holders Owning or Holding 1 Percent or more of Total Amount of Bonds, Mortgages, or Other Securities. If none, check box → ☐ None

Full Name	Complete Mailing Address
NA	

12. Tax Status (For completion by nonprofit organizations authorized to mail at nonprofit rates) (Check one)
The purpose, function, and nonprofit status of this organization and the exempt status for federal income tax purposes:
[X] Has Not changed During Preceding 12 Months
[ ] Has Changed During Preceding 12 Months (Publisher must submit explanation of change with this statement below)

PS Form 3526, July 2014

13. Publication Title			14. Issue Date for Circulation Data Below	
CLINICS IN SPORTS MEDICINE			October 2026	
15.	**Extent and Nature of Circulation**		**Average No. Copies Each Issue During Preceding 12 Months**	**No. Copies of Single Issue Published Nearest to filing Date**
a. Total Number of Copies (Net press run)			115	112
b. Paid and/or Requested Circulation	(1)	Mailed Outside-County Paid Subscriptions Stated on PS Form 3541 (Include paid distribution above nominal rate, advertiser's proof copies, and exchange copies)	67	72
	(2)	Mailed In-County Paid Subscriptions Stated on PS Form 3541 (Include paid distribution above nominal rate, advertiser's proof copies, and exchange copies)	0	0
	(3)	Paid Distribution Outside the Mails Including Sales Through Dealers and Carriers, Street Vendors, Counter Sales ,and Other Paid Distribution Ouside USPS	27	21
	(4)	Paid Distribution by Other Classes of Mail Through the USPS (e.g. First-Class Mail)	14	12
c. Total Paid Distribution [Sum of 15b. (1), (2), (3), and (4)] ▶			108	105
d. Free or Nominal Rate Distribution (By Mail and Outside the Mail)	(1)	Free or Nominal Rate Outside-County Copies Included on PS Form 3541	6	6
	(2)	Free or Nominal In-County Copies Included on PS Form 3541	0	0
	(3)	Free or Nominal Rate Copies Mailed at Other Classes Through the USPS (e.g. First-Class Mail)	0	0
	(4)	Free or Nominal Rate Distribution Outside the Mail (Carriers or other means)	1	1
e. Total Free or Nominal Rate Distribution (Sum of 15d. (1), (2), (3) and (4)) ▶			7	7
f. Total Distribution (Sum of 15c. and 15e.) ▶			115	112
g. Copies not Distributed (See Instructions to Publishers #4 (page #3))			0	0
h. Total (Sum of 15f. and g.) ▶			115	112
i. Percent Paid (15c. Divided by 15f. Times 100) ▶			93.91%	93.75%

* if you are claiming electronic copies, go to line 16 on page 3. If you are not claiming electronic copies, skip to line 17 on page 3.

16. Electronic copy Circulation		
If present, check box →		
a. Paid Electronic Copies		
b. Total Paid Print Copies (Line 15c) + Paid Electronic Copies (Line 16a) ▶	108	105
c. Total Print Distribution (Line 15f) + Paid Electronic Copies (Line 16a) ▶	115	112
d. Percentage Paid (Both Print & Electronic Copies (16b divided bt 16c x 100) ▶	93.91%	93.75%

[X] I certify that 50% of all my distribution copies (electronic and Print) are paid above a nominal price

17. Publication of Statement of Ownership
[X] Publication required. Will be printed in the **October 2026** issue of this publication. [ ] Publication not required

18. Signature and Title of Editor, Publisher, Business Manager, or Owner	Title	Date
Mohana Priya Damodharan	**Distribution Controller**	8/21/2026

I certify that all information furnished on this form is true and complete. I understand that anyone who furnishes false or misleading information on this form or who omits material or information requested on the form may be subject to criminal sanctions (including fines and imprisonment) and/or civil sanctions (including civil penalties)

PS Form **3526**, July 2014

9780443415869